Hairstyles and Fashion

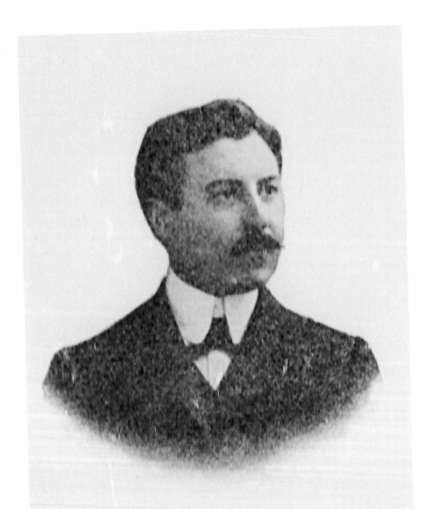

E. LONG

DRESS, BODY, CULTURE

Hairstyles and Fashion
A Hairdresser's History of Paris, 1910–1920

Edited with an introduction by

Steven Zdatny

Oxford • New York

First published in 1999 by
Berg
Editorial offices:
150 Cowley Road, Oxford, OX4 1JJ, UK
70 Washington Square South, New York, NY 10012, USA

Berg is an imprint of Oxford International Publishers Ltd.

Library of Congress Cataloging-in-Publication Data
A catalog record for this book is available from the Library of Congress.

British Library Cataloguing-in-Publication Data
A catalogue record for this book is available from the British Library.

ISBN   1 85973 217 8 (Cloth)
       1 85973 222 4 (Paper)

Typeset by JS Typesetting, Wellingborough, Northants.
Printed in the United Kingdom by Biddles Ltd, Guildford and King's Lynn.

Contents

Acknowledgements

I would like to thank the kind people at the Fédération Nationale de la Coiffure in Paris – president Pierre Séassari, general secretary Robert Maréchal, and Mme. Benoît – for welcoming me to their wonderful library. It was there that I discovered Long's marvelous epistles. A historian's work is impossible, of course, without financial assistance, for which I owe thanks to the Council for International Exchange of Scholars, the National Endowment for the Humanities, Augustana College, and West Virginia University. Kathryn Earle has been an encouraging and generous editor. Finally, I thank Edward McNally for his photography, hospitality, and friendship, as well as Sophie Zdatny, for her editing and loving indulgence. This book is dedicated to Jack E. Reece, a man of singular intelligence and integrity.

Steven Zdatny

Introduction *

It would make an interesting and useful assignment to ask students to choose some object of material culture and to write a brief history of it. Virtually any object would do: beds, clothes, cooking implements, washing facilities, and so on. Each of these would lead inevitably to a broader study of cultural practices: beds, for example, to a history of sleep; clothes to a study of fashion, gender, industry; etc. Students would of necessity pose fundamental and incisive questions about the past. How did people sleep? On what? With whom and for how long? How did people wash themselves? How often? Did they use soap? Did they wash everywhere or only in certain spots? Did they care about comfort and smell in the way that we do? Did they associate hygiene with health or even virtue? It seems clear that, in wide perspective or narrow, over the long term or the short, such an assignment would focus students on the most fundamental historical matter: what did it mean to be human in the past?

In fact, whatever they ask their students to do, historians have themselves been engaging in exactly this sort of research. Look at the growing historical literature about material culture and cultural history. The past twenty-or-so years have seen the publication of histories of smell, food, books, table manners, fashions, sex and sexuality, cafés, automobiles, and even pet-keeping.[1] Recently, the production of such inquiries has accelerated, with

---

*Throughout, I have tried to stay as close to Long's text as I could. While I have corrected some of the inconsistencies in his usage, I have left others as they were, and I have retained almost all of the original spelling.

1. Alain Corbin, *The Foul and the Fragrant: Odor and the French Social Imagination* (Cambridge MA: Harvard U. Press, 1986); Roger Chartier, *The Cultural Origins of the French Revolution* (Durham NC: Duke U. Press, 1991); Robert Darnton, *The Great Cat Massacre and Other Episodes in French Cultural History* (New York: Basic Books, 1984); W. Scott Haine, *The World of the Paris Café: Sociability Among the French Working Class, 1789–1914* (Baltimore: Johns Hopkins U. Press, 1996; Kathleen Kete, *The Beast in the Boudoir: Petkeeping in Nineteenth-Century Paris* (Berkeley: U. of California Press, 1994); Claudine Marenco, *Manières de table, modèles de moeurs, 17ème–20ème siècle* (Paris: Editions de l'ENS-Cachan, 1992); Michael B. Miller, *The Bon Marché: Bourgeois Culture and the Department Store, 1869–1920* (Princeton: Princeton U. Press, 1981); Philippe Perrot, *Fashioning the Bourgeoisie: A History of Clothing in the Nineteenth Century* (Princeton: Princeton U. Press,

studies of bicycles, home appliances, vacations, and movies beginning to appear in print.[2] Each object, each practice provides its own 'privileged site' for examining broader historical developments.

It is the first premise of this collection that one of those privileged sites sits on the top of our heads. Think of the questions to be asked. How is hair arranged? Is it left long or cut short? How often is it washed? Do people take care of their hair at home, or do they go to a salon? How much do they pay? Do the majority of women have their hair 'done' or only the privileged? The way a society deals with hair has a lot to tell us about its structures, its wealth and its values. Hair, the anthropologists might say, is good for thinking – thinking about consumer habits and technology, about notions of fashion and cleanliness, about changing ideals of femininity and the social order.

The second premise is that students derive special value from reading primary sources. Listening directly to the voice of the past they discover unfamiliar attitudes and preoccupations and hear the language in a different rhythm. Primary sources, especially such rich and literate ones as Long's essays, give students of history access to the past in way that even the best analytical and predigested treatments cannot.

The document that follows is edited from a long series of brief articles written by Emile Long, a French hairdresser, for his English colleagues. These appeared continuously from 1910 to 1920, in English, in a monthly supplement to the trade publication, the *Hairdressers' Weekly Journal*. Long's purpose in writing was to inform English coiffeurs about the goings on in the world of fashion and hairdressing in France, especially in Paris, the acknowledged capital of style and taste. And his readers must have welcomed the respite from the *Supplement*'s regular diet of reports on ringworm, eczema, and the other unappealing staples of the hairdressers' trade. Each of Long's

---

1994); Kristin Ross, *Fast Cars, Clean Bodies: Decolonization and the Reordering of French Culture* (Cambridge MA: MIT Press, 1995); Wolfgang Schivelbusch, *Tastes of Paradise: A Social History of Spices, Stimulants, and Intoxicants* (New York: Vintage, 1992); Rosalind Williams, *Dream Worlds: Mass consumption in Late Nineteenth-Century France* (Berkeley: U. of California Press, 1982). For the book that in many ways opened up this area of inquiry, see Norbert Elias, *The Civilizing Process, Vol. I: The History of Manners* (New York: Pantheon, 1978).

2. See, for example, Leo Charney and Vanessa R. Schwartz, eds., *Cinema and the Invention of Modern Life* (Berkeley: U. of California Press, 1995); Ellen Furlough, 'Packaging Pleasures: Club Méditerranée and French Consumer Culture, 1950–1968,' *French Historical Studies* (Spring 1993): 65–81. For a sample of the current interest in this sort of history, look at the programs for recent meetings of the Society for French Historical Studies or the *Proceedings of the Meetings of the Western Society for French History*.

articles examined some aspect of the art and business of coiffure. Usually the two aspects were combined, as Long described the ebb and flow of particular vogues in the context of coiffeurs' need to coax profit out of women's desire to be stylish.

Long was no social critic, but he had a powerful professional conscience and this made him a keen observer of the world around him. This enables him to offer the reader a relatively rare treat: not the cold, backward gaze of the historian but the involved, spontaneous, and authentic glance of the participant – a personal cultural history of the world's most fashionable city in a period that stretches from the end of the Belle Epoque, through the First World War, and into the opening year of the 'roaring twenties'. In this respect, Long's essays resemble such earlier testimonies as those of the eighteenth-century *boulevardier*, Restif de la Bretonne, and the nineteenth-century *compagnon*, Agricol Perdiguier.[3] Not many such documents are available to the general reader, which is the principal value of these pieces almost ninety years on.

The articles themselves comprise a history of hairstyles that takes its place within the larger history of fashion, an expanding field of study that has opened rich new perspectives on general developments. Once upon a time, fashion was outside the ken of most historians. What was written about it came in the form of memoirs by – or puffy biographies of – its significant figures.[4] Clothes themselves remained the more or less exclusive province of fashion historians and glossy catalogues. Lately, however, the increasing interest in things cultural has pulled fashion into the historical mainstream. Drawing on the classical sociological work of Thorsten Veblen and Georg Simmel, scholars have looked at the operation of fashion in society, the

3. Rétif de la Bretonne, *Les nuits de Paris ou le spectateur nocturne* (Paris, 1788); Agricol Perdiguier, *Mémoirs d'un compagnon* (Moulins: Editions des Cahiers du Centre, 1914).
4. For example, Pierre Balmain, *My Years and Seasons* (Garden City, NY: Doubleday and Co., 1965); Paul Poiret, *King of Fashion: The Autobiography of Paul Poiret* (Philadelphia and London: Lippencott, 1931); René Rambaud, *Les fugitives. Précis anécdotiques et historique des coiffures féminines à travers les âges, des Egyptiens à 1945* (Paris: René Rambaud, 1947); Stéphane (Coiffeur de Sa Majesté la Reine Elizabeth de Belgique) *L'art de la coiffure féminine. Son histoire à travers les siècles* (Paris: Editions de La Coiffure de Paris, 1932). Coco Chanel, the woman who put *les françaises* in trousers and sweaters, was a favorite subject. See Edmonde Charles-Roux, *L'irrégulière, ou mon itinéraire Chanel* (Paris: Grasset, 1974); Marylène Delbourg-Delphis, *Le chic et le look: histoire de la mode féminine et des moeurs de 1850 à nos jours* (Paris: Hachette, 1981); Pierre Galant, *Les années Chanel* (Paris: Editions Pierre Charron et Mercure de France, 1972); Marcel Haedrich, *Coco Chanel Secrète* (Paris: Editions Robert Lafont, 1971); Alice Mackrell, *Coco Chanel* (New York: Holmes and Meier, 1992).

'fashion system.' A new approach, derived principally from the methods of literary criticism, has directed researchers' attention to the clothes themselves, which – considered as a sort of 'text,' like a novel or painting – can be read and 'deconstructed.'[5]

Long himself was no theorist, but he had his own notions of what made the wheel of fashion spin – part Simmel, part Veblen, part Stuart Ewen and Naomi Wolf.[6] He seems to have believed that fashion originates in women's natural desires – 'the coquettish instinct of the primitive and barbarous races'[7] – stirred up to a passion by manufacturers' ability to massage and exploit these desires, driven forward (or sometimes backward) by an obsession for 'distinction,' and spread across society by the masses' attempts to ape the élites. On the whole, he thought of fashion as a force of nature, transhistorical, an unobjectionable and even benign process. Over the fashions themselves, various trades exerted more or less control: *couturiers* more than hat-shapers, hat-shapers more than milliners, milliners more than hairdressers; and above them all, the tyranny of feminine caprice.

However they interpret it, historians all concede that fashion is thick with historical and sociological meaning. In particular, it has taught us a lot about gender; that is, about the way ideals of masculinity and femininity are produced and disseminated – why, for example, modern Western women wear high heels and spend so much money on cosmetics.[8] Beyond gender, studies of the manufacture and retailing of fashion, especially of its role in maintaining high levels of consumer demand, have added to our under-

5. Georg Simmel, 'Fashion,' *The American Journal of Sociology* (May 1957), pp. 541-558; Thorsten Veblen, *The Theory of the Leisure Class: An Economic Study of Institutions* (Boston: Houghten Mifflin, 1973). On the semiotic approach to fashion, see Roland Barthes, *The Fashion System* (New York: Hill & Wang, 1983).

6. Stuart Ewen, *Captains of Consciousness: Advertising and the Social Roots of Consumer Culture* (New York: McGraw Hill, 1976); and Ewen, *Channels of Desire: Mass Images and the Shaping of American Consciousness* (Minneapolis: U. of Minnesota Press, 1992); Naomi Wolf, *The Beauty Myth: How Images of Beauty are Used Against Women* (New York: William Morrow & Co., 1991).

7. *Hairdressers' Weekly Journal. Supplement* (Hereafter *HWJS*), May 1913.

8. Lois Banner, *American Beauty* (New York: Alfred A. Knopf, 1983); Shari Benstock and Suzanne Ferriss, eds. *On Fashion* (New Brunswick NJ: Rutgers U. Press, 1994); Jane Gaines and Charlotte Herzog, eds., *Fabrications: Costume and the Female Body* (New York: Routledge, 1990); Susan Kingsley Kent, *Making Peace: The Reconstruction of Gender in Interwar Britain* (Princeton: Princeton U. Press, 1993); Kathy Peiss, 'Culture de masse et divisions sociales: le cas de l'industrie américaine des cosmétiques,' *Le Mouvement Social* 152 (July–September 1990), pp. 7–30; Mary Lou Roberts, *Civilization Without Sexes: Reconstructing Gender in Postwar France, 1917–1927* (Chicago: U. of Chicago Press, 1994); Elizabeth Wilson, *Adorned in Dreams: Fashion and Modernity* (Berkeley: University of California Press, 1985).

standing of the operation of the contemporary consumer economy.[9]

It is here, where marketing meets mass consumption, that fashion links gender to capitalism, precisely because some versions of femininity are better for business than others. While there may be no over-arching capitalist conspiracy to produce Women Who Shop, modern society is clearly full of messages that encourage women to define themselves through the things they wear. Fashion in this sense belongs not only to culture and economics, but to politics.[10]

By the time the *Hairdressers' Weekly Journal* began to publish his essays in 1910, Emile Long had already established himself among the handful of leading Paris hairdressers. He carried an impeccable pedigree, as protégé of the legendary Marcel Grateau, creator of the so-called 'Marcel' wave (see below), and was the perfect candidate to write for an English audience. Long had lived and worked in London around the turn of the century – he had even introduced Marcel to his English confreres – and was therefore familiar with the London fashion scene.[11]

Long revealed himself in these pages to be a man of varied interests and extraordinary energy. In addition to his work on the fashionable heads of Paris, he served as the general secretary of the profession's most élite club, the Institut des Coiffeurs de Dames, which listed as its headquarters Long's elegant salon on the rue de Moscou, in the Saint-Lazare quarter of the chic Eighth arrondissement. He even found time to teach a few classes in *ondulation* (hair waving) at the École Parisienne de la Coiffure, the training facilities run by the hairdressing workers union. At the same time as he was sending his monthly contributions to the *Hairdressers' Weekly Journal*, Long also founded and wrote for the French trade weekly, the *Capilartiste*, and edited the fashion review, *Paris-Coiffures*, where his sketches helped coiffeurs and their clients stay *au courant* with the latest hairstyles.

9. Judith Coffin, *The Politics of Women's Work: The Paris Garment Trades, 1750–1915* (Princeton: Princeton U. Press, 1996); Nancy L. Green, 'Art and Industry: The Language of Modernization in the Production of Fashion,' *French Historical Studies* 18 (Spring 1994), pp. 722–48, and Green, *Ready-to-Wear, Ready-to-Work: A Century of Industry and Immigrants in Paris and New York* (Durham: Duke U. Press, 1997; Lori Ann Loeb, *Consuming Angels: Advertising and Victorian Women* (New York: Oxford U. Press, 1994); Kathy Peiss, 'Industry and the Cultural construction of Gender,' *Genders* 7 (Spring 1990), pp. 143–69.

10. Richard Butsch, ed. *For Fun and Profit: The Transformation of Leisure into Profit* (Philadelphia: Temple University Press, 1990); Stuart Ewen, *All Consuming Images: The Politics of Style in Contemporary Culture* (New York: Basic Books, 1988); Alan Tomlinson, ed., *Consumption, Identity, and Style: Marketing, Meanings and the Packaging of Pleasure* (London: Routledge, 1990).

11. Paul Gerbod, *Histoire de la Coiffure et des Coiffeurs* (Paris: Larousse, 1995), p. 211.

As far as his colleagues were concerned, Long probably made his most important contribution to the profession when he published the *Traité d'Ondulation*, which the *Hairdressers' Weekly Journal* later serialized as 'A Complete Illustrated Treatise on Hair Waving.'[12] In the *Traité* Long explained and illustrated the fabulous techniques of his mentor, Marcel Grateau, inventor of the eponymous 'Marcel wave.' For twenty years Marcel had refused to divulge the technique that was making him so rich. But Marcel's retirement in 1907 authorized Long to do so. That he so blithely gave away his patron's jealously guarded and highly remunerative secrets was further proof of Long's devotion to his profession.

The impulse that drove these articles was Long's pursuit of fashion and the fashionable. He observed them strolling the *grands boulevards*. He accompanied them to the opera and to the races at Auteuil and Longchamps. He watched them at the *grandes soirées* and *travesties* (costume balls), where the *beau monde* was at its most outrageous. Long peeked into the showrooms of the most *à la mode* couturiers and modistes, to which his own celebrity gave him entrée. In August, when the Paris 'seasons' were finished and *le tout Paris* abandoned the hot city, Long followed them to the Channel resorts of Deauville and Trouville.

For it was not only in the capital that fashionable reputations were made. Alexandre, the most celebrated coiffeur of the post-Second World War era, who counted among his clients Grace Kelly and Elizabeth Taylor, was 'discovered' in Cannes, just after the war, by the Duchess of Windsor, who brought him to Paris a couple of years later.[13] However, the most famous instance of fame won at the seashore was probably that of Alexandre's patron, the incomparable Antoine 'de Paris', who appeared throughout Long's articles as one of the radical 'young lions' of the hairdressing profession. Born Antek Cierplikowski, in Siedradz, Poland, Antoine learned his trade and developed his genius in Łòdz, an apprentice to his uncle. The ambitious young coiffeur left Poland and arrived in Paris in 1901. His first position brought him to the salon of the Galeries Lafayette department store, but he soon began to work the 'season' in Deauville as well.

There, in the summer of 1904, Antoine got his big break. In his auto-biography Antoine recalls his opportunity to dress the hair of Lily de Moure, mistress of a Prince of the Blood, for an evening in Deauville Society. Poor Mlle de Moure suffered a *crise*, however, when she somehow lost the hat

---

12. Emile Long, *Traité complet et illustré de l'ondulation artificielle des cheveux* (Paris: Albert Brunet, 1909).

13. On Alexandre and the Duchess of Windsor see Gisèle d'Assailly, *Fards et Beauté. Ou l'éternel féminin* (Paris: Hachette, 1958), pp. 259–65.

that was to have finished her extraordinary toilette. Soothing her and giving her courage, Antoine convinced de Moure that she could take the unheard of step of going hatless on such an occasion, and he set about creating a suitably fabulous coiffure. The Prince himself was sitting admiringly in the boudoir when a maid arrived with the missing hat. But Antoine did not want his *chef d'oeuvre* ruined, and he prevailed upon de Moure to leave it home and go out *sans chapeau*. The bareheaded Lily de Moure on the arm of a prince caused a sensation, and the next morning a line of fashionable ladies gathered at the door of the Maison Decoux, where Antoine worked, begging to be served by 'le petit rousse' (the 'little Russian' – *sic*). Whether the tale is apocryphal or not – and Antoine was a notorious self promoter – it illustrates the unpredictable way in which styles were made and stars born.[14]

Long does not retell the story of Antoine's breakthrough, which took place several years before he began to write for the *Hairdressers' Weekly Journal*. Yet his own articles are full of similar stories about the rich and famous, which add up to a sort of anecdotal archeology of fashion. However, business, not amusement, was the point of these essays. In eleven years of reporting from the battle front of fashion, Long never strayed far from his chief preoccupation: how were women wearing their hair, and how might hairdressers profit from it?

Our tour of fashion and culture begins in 1910, at the height of the Belle Epoque. Paris was the center of *civilisation* – and not only in fashion, where the houses of Lanvin, Poiret, and Worth set the pace for the rest of the world. Picasso was painting in the French capital. So were Kandinsky, Chagall, Braque, Matisse, and others. Proust was writing, Stravinsky composing. A young Maurice Chevalier, alongside his actress girlfriend, Mistinguett, was beginning to make his career in French vaudeville. In the evenings, the cultural avant garde might be seen at the Chat Noir or the Moulin Rouge, surrounded by bourgeois, *demi-mondaines*, and a crowd of curious tourists.[15] More conventional members of fashionable society amused themselves at great parties and masked balls.

---

14. On Antoine see Antoine, *J'ai coiffé le monde entier* (Paris: La Table Ronde, 1963); Gerbod, *Histoire*, p. 202; Charles Graves, *Devotion to Beauty: The Antoine Story* (London: Jarrold's, 1962); Guillaume, *Guillaume raconte . . . la coiffure et ses métamorphoses* (Argenton-sur-Creuse: Imprimerie de l'Indre, 1982), p. 19; Catherine Lebas and Annie Jacques, *La coiffure en France du Moyen Age à nos jours* (Paris: Delmas International, 1979), p. 278.

15. Charles Rearick, *Pleasures of the Belle Epoque: Entertainment and Festivity in Turn-of-the-Century France* (New Haven: Yale U. Press, 1985); Deborah L. Silverman, *Art Nouveau in Fin-de-Siècle France* (Berkeley: U. of California Press, 1989); Roger Shattuck, *The Banquet Years: The Origins of the Avant-Garde in France, 1885 to World War I* (New York: Vintage, 1968).

Long's narrative continues through the war, when the guns of August put an end to this frothy cultural life, or at least forced it into embarrassed restraint, and into the postwar period, in an atmosphere redolent with the cultural pessimism of Dada and the early fascism of writers like Drieu la Rochelle.[16] But victorious France was also a country *folle* with the grandeur and relief of victory, just beginning to vibrate with a new culture of film, cars, and youth.

As we read Long's reports from Paris, the first thing we see – because it is the first thing he saw – is the parade of hairstyles stretching from Edwardian *grandes dames* to postwar *garçonnes*, accompanied always by Long's brilliant illustrations. His initial report, in January 1910, set the tone for the rest. In it he took up the matter of the disastrous 'turban' look and the 'cocoanut' coiffure, which had depressed the demand for waves and badly hurt hairdressers' business. In subsequent articles we observe the passing of the 'Clown,' the Pyramid,' the 'Casque,' and the 'Phrygian Bonnet,' with its playful allusion to the bloody days of the French Revolution. Some women began to sport curls, or coiffures with double partings; others dared to uncover their ears.[17] Even the War could not halt the march of women's hairstyles. In 1916, the highly ornamental '1830s' style was popular. Two-and-a-half years later, as the Allies breached the Hindenburg Line, the 'Bonnet Japonnais' was the *mode du jour*. With the Armistice, the pace of fashion began once more to accelerate. At postwar *soirées* and victory balls Long discovered (to his horror) hair styled *à la Chinoise* – pulled back straight away from the face and fashioned in a ponytail – *à l'Egyptienne*, *à la Grecque*, and in the manner of the 'Dog's Ear,' to mention only those coiffures prominent enough to earn a moniker. The wheel of fashion never ceased to turn, mixing the old with the new, the sublime with the ridiculous.

Each *mode* entailed some change in the shape and composition of the hair; each presented Long and his colleagues with the same basic challenge: how to turn it to account. Styles became straighter or wavier, chignons rose and fell between the nape of the neck and the crown of the head. Some required large postiches, some small, others none at all. Moreover, at any one time, French women were wearing many different hairstyles, and public taste was

16. Modris Ecksteins, *Rites of Spring: The Great War and the Birth of the Modern Age* (Boston: Houghton Mifflin, 1989).

17. For interesting discussions of prewar hairstyles see the seminar on the history of coiffure, conducted by Henri Lecoq and reproduced in the *Ouvrier Coiffeur*, May 1913, available in the the Archives Nationales [hereafter AN], Paris, F⁷ 13693, dossier 'Coiffeurs, 1913'; Jane Mulvagh, *Vogue's History of Twentieth-Century Fashion* (London: Viking, 1988); and the review of twenty years of fashion in *Vogue* magazine, September 1924, pp. 16–7 (all citations refer to the French Edition).

forever in motion. In the fall of 1909, the esteemed *coiffeur-posticheur*, Crozier-Noirat, writing in the trade journal, *La Coiffure de Paris*, noted that the *mode à la Belle Poule* ('beautiful hen' style) worn by the Countess G. was all the rage in Paris, but he cautioned readers that it was impossible to predict what would be the 'dernier cri' (last word) next year.

Long began his series in January 1910 with a cautionary tale about Mme Letellier, 'the handsomest woman in Paris,' whose portraits came near to ruining the hairdressing profession. In the summer of 1907 at Trouville, Letellier's portrait had been painted by a member of what Long called the 'modern school.' These painters, according to Long, hated heavily waved hair because they lacked the talent and patience to paint the necessary detail. The portrait of Mme. Letellier therefore showed her with straight hair. This artistic short cut subsequently became a convention when the celebrated artist, Hellenu, began to paint portraits of many of France's most fashionable young women – once again, with absolutely straight hair, although all of them wore wavy coiffures. Life soon came to imitate art as the fashion magazine, *Femina*, following Hellenu, spread the impression among, first, 'the upper circle,' and, later, the 'great public . . . that it was not necessary to wave so much – that, in fact, waving was no longer the fashion.' It was this impression, so circuitously produced, that led to the popularity of the 'turban headdress' and other straight styles, thus suppressing the lucrative 'Marcel' wave that had dominated styles and made coiffeurs happy for thirty years.[18]

The genesis of the 'turban' illustrates a critical principle of fashion: while the outlines of fashion were to some degree determined by technological possibilities and the historical moment, in a more immediate way, the kingdom of fashion was ruled by serendipity. Consider what Long learned in October 1910, when he visited the leading Parisian *modistes* (milliners), in the company of his friend, M. Perrin, one of the most 'eminent' of their number. Long sought out the milliners because he believed they had learned to control public taste and thereby to assure their prosperity. He wanted to discover how. He also understood that, from season to season and for obvious reasons, hats set the effective limits for hairstyles. Hairdressers therefore could profit from knowing what the milliners had in store.

Long and Perrin approached the capital's greatest *modistes* and asked what they were preparing for the coming season. The reply they received every-where was 'toques – toques in velvet and furs of all kinds.'[19] 'Why,' Long asked, 'are you giving a preference to toques?' No doubt he expected an answer that combined sociological insight and marketing genius. What he

---

18. *HWJS*, 1 January 1910.
19. A toque is a brimless, shapeless hat, like a chef's hat.

got was something else. 'We do not make toques out of preference,' the *grands modistes* told him, 'but simply because our hat shapers have been on strike for four months and we cannot procure felt shapes.' So much for a semiotics of hat styles.

Presumably, fashionable parisiennes were all wearing toques in the coming months, but that cannot be taken for granted. For if there is one thing Long had discovered in his career, it was that customers did not always do as they were bidden. Almost inevitably, Long wrote, women wanted one thing for their hair and coiffeurs another, and in this basic truth lay a perpetual source of conflict between coiffeurs and their clients. It was only every fifteen or twenty years, he added, when voluminous and complex coiffures came into fashion, that this tension subsided for a time.[20] As a rule, Long counseled, this conflict was best resolved through accommodation. Coiffeurs should cede to customers' wishes, even if those wishes did not correspond to hair-dressers' best interests. Smaller profits, he reasoned, were better than fewer customers, and a woman who did not get what she wanted from one coiffeur would certainly leave him for another.

Yet Long could never completely convince himself that it was impossible to guide the public's inclinations, and he continued to believe that others in the fashion industry – *couturiers* and *modistes* especially – were able to nudge them in profitable directions. These *marchandes de modes*, Long wrote enviously, were exceedingly clever at 'creating business by continually varying their creations and making their seductiveness overpowering.' Given that hairdressers stood to profit handsomely from the 'right' hairstyles and lose considerably from the 'wrong' ones, it made sense for them to organize so as to push women's modish instincts along the proper course. This motive lay behind the formation of what Long called the Fashion Committee of Parisian *hauts coiffeurs*. The Fashion Committee aimed to impose discipline on the profession, to encourage its members to set an example by exhibiting only the most lucrative styles. To this end, the Committee recommended each month the coiffures that all hairdressers should display in their store windows – the more effectively to influence both clients and passersby.

On the other hand, while Long himself belonged to the Fashion Committee and agreed that the trade needed more coordination and discipline, he never fully believed it would succeed. For one thing, Long doubted that women's preferences could be manipulated so easily. Fashion was powerful and capricious: 'We can no more resist the on-coming of Fashion,' he wrote, 'than we can stop the impetuous torrent of a mighty river.'[21] It could not be prescribed,

20. *HWJS*, July 1911.
21. *HWJS*, November 1910.

'only seized at the moment of its appearance.' For another, with so many coiffeurs at work, the profession was incorrigibly 'anarchic.' Hairdressing had its leading figures. Yet they were in no position to govern coiffure in the way that powerful manufacturers like Worth, Lanvin, Paquin, and Poiret could dominate *couture*. Indeed, the Fashion Committee, even when it decided to push a certain style, could hardly count on the cooperation of its own members. In the fall of 1911, for example, Long reported that the Committee was almost unanimous 'in favor of the low chignon, combined with locks of false hair for day wear and curls on the neck for the evening.' However, as he toured the city's salons he discovered that not one member of the Committee was exhibiting the styles 'which the committee wishes to impose on the bulk of their colleagues.'[22]

Anarchy was compounded by philosophical and artistic differences. The élite of the profession were split between two groups, whom Long called 'classicists' and 'modernists.' The differences between them offer another lesson in audacity, marketing, and popular taste. By 'classicists' Long indicated the tradition-bound doyens of *haute coiffure*, who favored proportionally modest coiffures and who, in Long's words, modeled 'their ideas and methods on judgment and good taste.' In contrast, the 'modernists' were a 'daringly enterprising' group of young men who desired 'radical changes' in hairstyles. Their number included important figures like Antoine, renown for his dramatic cuts and 'Bulgarian' colors, and François, famous for his outsized postiches.

The 'classicists' had more fixed notions about what was becoming and appropriate on a woman's head and generally refused to style hair in ways that offended their inbred sense of beauty. The 'modernists' brought fewer preconceptions to their art. They were willing to satisfy, even to encourage, any public whim, however outlandish. Long's aesthetic sympathies generally lay with 'classicists,' whose training he shared, and he often disapproved of the 'modernists'' work. In March 1912 Long witnessed a demonstration by François, the most prominent of the avant garde. He found the young man's hairstyles excessively simple, 'destitute of knots, curls, interlacings and all kinds of details' and on the whole 'lacking in prettiness, not practical or becoming . . . likened . . . to a Dervish's bonnet, a bundle of hay, and so on.'

At the same time as he failed to appreciate their art, however, Long admired the 'modernists'' commercial acuity. They had their manicured fingers on the public pulse to a much greater degree than their competitors. The 'modernists' succeeded largely by acceding to their clients' desires, and Long had to

---

22. *HWJS*, November 1911 and February 1912.

admit that their openness and innovation presented coiffeurs with more profitable opportunities than the stodginess of the 'classicists.' By the early 1920s, propelled by the increasing influence of young women on contemporary fashion, 'modern' styles had completely eclipsed 'classical' ones.

If coiffeurs quarreled among themselves over artistic values and business strategy, they also experienced more fundamental and serious clashes of interest with other elements of the fashion industry. In 1919, for example, Long described a conflict that pitted hairdressers against the so-called drapery establishments, who were heavily promoting ribbons. 'Nowadays in Paris,' wrote Long with some disgust, 'even the meanest midinette or milliner's assistant sports her little bit of ribbon.'[23] The problem was that women tended to use ribbon to replace the more expensive items with which coiffeurs used to dress their hair. Long alluded to similar friction between ladies' hairdressers and *couturiers*. Having entrée to the most exclusive showrooms, Long found that the great couturiers always required their *mannequins* to wear smallish, simple hairstyles. No doubt the *couturiers* did not want to detract from the effect of their clothes. Nevertheless, Long noted, it sent clients the wrong message about fashionable hair.[24]

Couturiers and ribbon-makers aside, coiffeurs experienced their most intimate and combative relationship with the milliners, as those who dressed hair battled those who covered it up. *Modistes* held most of the cards in this contest. They enjoyed a clear precedence over coiffures in the great chain of fashion being, largely because hats were not considered an optional accessory but were always worn on public occasions – witness the scandal caused by Mlle de Moure. Consequently, hairdressers' fortunes usually depended on hat styles, rather than the other way around. A pretty affair for the *modistes* might therefore be a disaster for coiffeurs. In February 1910, Long complained about 'gigantic, bell-shaped hats [*chapeaux cloches*] – the sort of extinguishers which envelope not only the hair but almost the whole of the head,' and which left hairdressers little to work with.

Attempts to smooth relations between these rival trades had some success. More critically, smaller hats came into fashion after 1913 and for many years thereafter, which eased hairdressers' anxiety. The principal exception to this trend was the vogue for the 'Bersagliere' – 'martial, befitting, and graceful' and with a wide brim – which flared briefly in the summer of 1915, after Italy entered the war on France's side.[25] Shrinking hats pleased coiffeurs well enough, but they were not good business for the *modistes*. They suggest,

23. *HWJS*, June 1919.
24. See, for example, *HWJS*, April 1911.
25. *HWJS*, August 1915.

moreover, that Long overestimated the milliners' ability to control popular taste, and that the same cultural forces favoring more comfortable clothes and shorter hair were also compelling milliners to produce less cumbersome hats.

Long worried about hats because they interfered directly with coiffeurs' ability to make money. Traditionally, ladies' hairdressers had earned their reputations and fortunes by weaving intricate patterns into a woman's hair and by placing in it any number of baubles and other items: flowers, combs, pearls, and fabrics. Thus, when Jourliac recommended the styles 'Directoire' and 'Empire modernisée' for 1909 and 1910, he imagined them full of postiches, chignons, plaits, and *torsades* (braids). *Vogue*, the toniest of women's magazines, described for its readers *coiffures du soir* replete with garlands of fruit and flowers, bands of gilded leaves, and thick satin ribbons.[26] The cost of such preparations was enormous. Historian Eugene Weber writes that at the summit of society, an actress, like Caroline Otéro, or a courtesan, like Liane de Pougy, might pay 900 or 1,600 francs for a ballgown – 'a good deal more,' he notes, 'than their maids' annual wages.'[27] The accompanying coiffure might cost almost as much.

Long's articles are full of discussions and illustrations of these various 'ornamental aids to coquetry and usefulness.' He described the interior pads that 'hold up' high coiffures, as well as the ribbons and combs that held them together. In March 1910, he informed his readers about the invention of the 'Marie-Louise' barrette, a brilliant little gadget to connect two bits of postiche. In May 1913, Long examined the new vogue for very long feathers, 'which would turn the last of the Redskins green with envy.' The taste for such *chachkas* came and went with the seasons; that for excessive plumage returned in 1919, when Long found himself sitting behind a woman at the theater: '[Her] feathers,' he told his readers, 'appear to come out of the ears, and the horizontal position makes them a source of annoyance to people sitting next to the wearer.' Long's illustration filled out the picture.[28]

Long thought this particular mode ridiculous, but he understood perfectly well that a coiffeur's prosperity depended exactly on the deployment of such knick-knacks. We need only compare the situation of *coiffeurs pour dames* to that of *coiffeurs pour hommes* (barbers). During the Belle Epoque, a barber would have had to trim thirty or thirty-five beards a day, at 20 centimes

---

26. For a lesson in wretched excess see *La Coiffure de Paris*, Oct.–Nov. 1909; *Journal de la Coiffure*, March 1902; A. Mallement, *Manuel de la Coiffure des Dames* (Paris: E. Robinet, 1898), p. 51; Rambaud, *Les fugitives*, p. 148; *Vogue*, 1 June 1921, pp. 3–5.

27. Eugen Weber, *France: Fin-de-Siècle* (Cambridge, MA: Harvard U. Press, 1986), p. 97.

28. *HWJS*, September 1919.

each, to produce eight and a half francs of income. Men's haircuts generally cost about 30 centimes, although smarter shops might charge as much as 50 centimes. If a *figaro* could talk his client into a *friction*, a bit of hair tonic, he would add another franc or so to his take, and he could usually count on a small *pourboire* (tip) dropped casually into the *tronc* (tip box) as the customer left – although the workers often complained that the employers kept most of this tip money for themselves. In any event, the miserable prices barbers charged for their services explain why they suffered some of the worst conditions of any workers in the capital, why wages were so low, hours so long, and days off so rare. Prices began to rise during the war – to 1 franc for a shave and 2 or 3 francs for a haircut, but this hardly threatened to make barbers rich.[29]

The lesson was clear: work alone could not provide hairdressers with a decent living, and this was true even for *coiffeurs pour dames*. Long reported in June 1917 that for a dressing at a down-market shop, a woman would pay 2 francs, waving included, which would require 30 to 45 minutes of work for the coiffeur or coiffeuse. This explains why Long paid relatively little attention to work and so much to commerce. For the opportunity to add a lot of value to a woman's head was precisely what saved ladies' hairdressers from the unfortunate lot of barbers. Consider the menu of decorations and treatments that a ladies' hairdresser of the Belle Epoque could offer his clients: Starting with 5 francs for a shampoo and 20 francs for a 'Marcel' wave, he could pile on combs, jewels, and postiches that might add hundreds of francs.

Although Long did not say it explicitly, all his readers would have understood that the *sine qua non* of a beautiful hairdo was long, luxurious hair. At the turn of the century, wrote Antoine, hair was judged by its length and weight. Most women never had their hair cut, and it was a proud mother, according to Antoine, who could say, 'My daughter is able to sit on her

---

29. For information on prices and working conditions see Archives de la Préfecture de Police, Paris, Bª1419, *Le Rappel*, 16 March 1900; AN F⁷ 13963, dossier Coiffeurs, 1914–1918; A Coffignon, *Les coulisses de la mode* (Paris: La Librairie Illustrée, 1888), pp. 19, 30; *La Coiffure de Paris*, January and June 1920; Richard Corson, *Fashions in Hair: The First Five Thousand Years* (London: Peter Owen, 1965), p. 561; Charles Desplanques, *Barbiers, perruquiers, coiffeurs* (Paris: Librairie Octave Doin, 1927), pp. 145, 237; *Journal de la Coiffure*, June 1902; Ministère du Commerce, de l'Industrie, des Postes et des Télégraphes. Office du Travail, *Les associations professionnelles ouvrières*, tome IV (Paris: Imprimerie Nationale, 1904), 'Coiffeurs de Paris,' p. 763; Ministère du Travail et de Prévoyance sociale. Statistique générale de la France, *Salaires et coûts d'existence à diverses époques, jusqu'en 1910* (Paris: Imprimerie Nationale, 1911), pp. 146–7.

hair.'[30] In fact, most *coiffeurs pour dames* probably had no idea how to use a scissors, being accustomed only to arranging and not to cutting hair. The voluminous and ornate styles of the day received such precious names as 'Queen of Spades' and 'Bird Charmer.'

Even the most exquisite ornaments and modern technology could not rescue a hairstyle made with thin, limp hair, and it was a fact that most women's hair lacked the qualities necessary to a first-class coiffure, but hairdressers had always been able to compensate for deficient nature through the manufacture and liberal use of postiches, pre-styled hairpieces. No weapon in a coiffeur's arsenal, thought Long, was more essential to art and to the bottom line. Postiche, at least before the coming of the permanent wave, was his principal source of added value, the item that lifted *coiffeurs pour dames* above their barbering colleagues. 'Postiche,' Long observed in July 1910, 'rids us of the slavery attached to continual shaving.'

The problem was that the demand for postiches fluctuated with the fashion of the moment. That demand had plunged in the 1880s and again around 1909 with the vogue for straight hair and the 'turban' look. Yet women's desire for postiches always seemed to return, and despite his perpetual worries, Long often reported a healthy market for them. In August 1913, Long wrote that the styles favored light but expensive postiches, whereas in June 1916 the new models exhibited by the Houses of Cuverville and Calou featured big postiches, some the size of full wigs. In November 1918, at the moment of the Armistice, Long told his readers that the postiche 'has acquired . . . a degree of perfection which can scarcely be surpassed, because it equals the highest natural qualities of artistic attractiveness.' Even the growing trend for short hair did not seem to kill women's appetite for postiches, which could serve both originality and convenience and which, according to *Vogue* magazine, could lend even the shortest cuts a 'dignité de circonstance' for the evening.[31]

One glance at the price of postiches would explain Long's enthusiasm. The most eminent coiffeurs were traditionally also the greatest artists of postiche, and the masterpiece they created for a client was often the most expensive item on her head. At the high end of the market, the creations of the great *maisons* of Cuverville, Calou, Jourliac, François, Croizier-Noirat, and Antoine would cost up to 500 francs – 'in the prettiest up-to-date tints, [more] if the hair is grey or of rare colour.' A step down the scale, a woman

---

30. Antoine, *J'ai coiffé*, p. 70. On the long styles of the era also see the illustrations in *Journal de la Coiffure*, March 1902; *Figaro-Modes*, January 1904; Gerbod, *Histoire*, p. 210; and *Vogue*, September 1924, p. 17.

31. See *Vogue*, July-December 1924, p. 52; *Coiffure et Modes*, April 1920.

could buy a postiche from Chez Mazy for between 250 and 400 francs. Even the far-from-élite D. Simon sold his postiches for up to 150 francs.[32]

Obviously, the majority of *françaises* could not afford these prices. Yet, by the end of 1918 Long estimated that 75 to 80 per cent of French women were wearing some sort of postiche. What this suggests is a considerable growth in the mass demand for stylish things. This both helped and hurt hairdressers. On the one hand, the 'vulgarization' of fashion brought millions of new customers to the *salons de coiffure*; on the other, increasing differentiation in the market often cost them old business. Long's meditations on this key development usually took the form of complaints that, at the bottom of the market, consumers were buying their postiches, not at the salon but from parfumeurs, haberdashers, and department stores, where a woman on a budget could buy mass-produced postiches at low prices – a textbook example of artisanal manufacture menaced by industrial production.

Long's business side found the ready-to-wear postiches from the trade houses and drapery establishments to be 'rather a convenient idea' for middle-class ladies, but the artist in him recoiled in horror from what he saw on the heads of the masses. Long described with obvious distaste the small, frizzy, wavy pieces bought by 'many coquettes possessing no personal taste and to whom it would be impossible to sell postiche of the latest design and make.' As for those who flooded the market with cheap postiches for sale through coiffeurs' competitors, Long condemned both their methods and effect. They used, he wrote, 'common hair' and harsh processes, such as glue diluted in boiling water. This inevitably produced hairpieces that kept their shape but looked terrible, and which, 'by their inartistic, inelegant and defective [qualities] create amongst the public a disgust for postiche work generally.'[33]

Postiche was not the only source of commercial profit for ladies' hairdressers at this time. Although Long paid less attention to hair coloring (*teinture*) than to postiche, his articles nonetheless chronicled its rising popularity among *parisiennes*. In the spring of 1912, at the races at Auteuil, Long noticed that mahogany-red and brown hair, made possible by the development of new black hennas, were replacing the blond hair that had previously been the vogue. The following summer he wrote that,

At one of our recent race meetings, which all the most fashionable people attend, the gay Parisians were able to admire two superb young ladies with remarkable toilettes and not less remarkable light grey hair under their black hats. As they

32. On the price of postiches see *La Coiffure de Paris*, January 1920; *HWJS*, November 1918; *La Mode Illustrée*, July 1921.

33. *HWJS*, October and December 1917.

had young faces the astonishment was general, but everybody agreed that they looked very nice, and, on the following day, all the papers announced this unforeseen event and commented favorably upon it.

On other occasions Long reported seeing less organic colors: blue, green, mauve – the so-called 'Bulgarian' colors made famous by Antoine – and remarked ghoulishly how well they went with fashionable dark hats and mourning veils.[34]

The expanding market for *teinture*, like that for postiche, pointed to changes in mores, markets, and demography. Hair coloring was an ancient practice, and it had been far from rare in nineteenth-century France.[35] Yet even in the Belle Epoque there remained something vaguely naughty about it. Add to this the fact that in an era of rudimentary chemistry, *teinture* could produce some unfortunate effects on hair and scalp. The actress, Caroline Otéro, was seriously burned in 1909 when several drops of the lotion she was pouring on her head came into contact with a hot-water heater.[36] The public prosecutor of the Seine Department registered 142 complaints relating to hair-coloring torts in 1902, and the fear of burns, rashes, and defoliation remained endemic.[37]

The status of *teinture* began to change dramatically in the twentieth century, pushed from two directions. First, dyes made from vegetable matter, especially henna, made hair coloring much less risky. At the same time, the rising 'cult of youth' made gray hair seem less inevitable. By 1920, coiffeur Raul Patois could write that sales of cheap dyes were five times greater than before the war: '*Teinture* is not the most agreeable work in the profession,' he added, 'but it is without comparison the most lucrative.[38]

The great pioneer of *teinture* was Eugène Schueller, the chemist who invented l'Oréal hair coloring in 1909. A brilliant chemist and restless entrepreneur, Schueller spent the next twenty years developing new products, building a fashion and publishing empire, and pouring millions of francs back into advertising and subsidies for the coiffeurs on his payroll. He was without question, from a commercial point of view, the most important single figure in the hairdressing profession up to the outbreak of the Second World

34. *HWJS*, April 1915.

35. See Theodore Zeldin, *France, 1848-1945. Vol. II: Intellect, Taste and Anxiety* (Oxford: Oxford U. Press, 1977), p. 441.

36. *Journal de la Coiffure*, February 1904; and reports of accidents in July and August 1903. See also the discussion in Georges-Lévy, *Hygiène du cuir chevelu et de la chevelure* (Paris: G. Doin, 1934), pp. 99–100.

37. *La Coiffure de Paris*, October–November 1909, p. 14.

38. *La Coiffure de Paris*, January 1920.

War, the basis of his fortune the safe, durable hair coloring he began to sell before World War I. L'Oréal became a rich and dependable source of income for thousands of coiffeurs.

The success of *teinture* was above all a triumph of technology, which was changing hairdressing as it was transforming all of society. Long's articles recognized only obliquely the impact of technology on hairdressers' lives. Normally preoccupied with day-to-day matters of style and business, they seldom dealt with larger historical issues. Yet the effect of technology was implicit in every matter Long discussed, from the development of public appetites to their satisfaction.

Envision the up-to-date hairdressing salon of 1920. Electric lamps lit the room. Along one wall sat marble-topped sinks, with hot running water. Down another ran a bank of hair dryers, powered by electricity or gas. (Antoine claimed to have been the first to install hair dryers in his luxurious salon on the rue Cambon, at the back of the Ritz Hotel, in 1905.)[39] Hanging on the wall, within arm's reach of the reclinable chairs, was the electric curling iron, which had come into the salons before the turn of the century and made much quicker work of the 'marcel.'[40] The new floor was laid with linoleum, easy to sweep and wash.[41]

Full of the gleaming tools of added value, the modern salon was a monument to the bright new age of fashionable consumption. More than that, its sinks, hot-water heaters, and shampoos for sale bore witness to one of the most momentous, if often overlooked, revolutions of the era: changing popular habits of personal hygiene. Antoine was among those seeking to change the habits of ladies of fashion, who had long considered shampooing 'inutile et humiliant.'[42] He told the following story. In 1904 he went to the residence of the Comtesse de Farge to dress her hair for a special occasion and was taken aback by the state of the Countess's hair, 'so greasy' he remembered, 'that one could have made a bad soup from it.' Antoine

39. Gas hair dryers came first. They were easier to use in that the hose carried no cumbersome attachments, as the electric dryers did. The electric dryers that followed were more expensive, yet they avoided the problem of carbon monoxide emissions that made the gas dryers dangerous. See M. Joyeux, 'Le gaz chez les coiffeurs: Ce qui nous amène à vous parler des salons de coiffure,' extrait du *Journal des Usines de Gaz*, 5–20 April 1936, pp. 5–8; and A. Spale, *Manuel du Coiffeur* (Paris: Librairie J.-B. Baillière et fils, 1933), pp. 119–20. Also, Antoine, *J'ai coiffé*, pp. 114–15.

40. Hairdresser and amateur historian René Rambaud wrote that the first French curling iron was introduced to France 1897, by Delot, two years after German and American versions of it: Rambaud, *Les fugitives*, p. 133.

41. C. Kauffmann and J. Barth, *Le livret du coiffeur. Technologie* (Paris: Librairie d'Enseignement Technique, 1923), p. 101.

42. Antoine, *J'ai coiffé*, pp. 92–3.

suggested strongly that he wash her hair before dressing it. The Countess was aghast. 'No,' she replied. 'Never. Understand that I *never* shampoo. *J'ai horreur de ça!*' Antoine shot back, 'The truth, Madame, is that I would not touch your hair in such a filthy state,' and he turned to leave, accompanied by a hail of insults 'that would have done credit to a fishmonger.'

Historian Eugen Weber has also noted the primitive state of the technology and culture of hygiene at the end of the nineteenth century. The scarcity of water in particular meant that 'washing was rare and bathing rarer.' 'In France,' Weber quoted Vacher de Lapouge, 'most women die without having once taken a bath.' The Comtesse de Pange recalled that:

> At seventeen, I had very long hair which, when loosened, wrapped around me like a mantle. But these beautiful tresses were never washed. They were stiff and filthy. The word shampoo was ignored. From time to time they rubbed my hair with quinine water.[43]

The point is clear. On the eve of the twentieth century, even privileged ladies of fashion mostly avoided washing their hair. How much less likely to shampoo were lower- and middle-class women, given the rarity and expense of hot water.

As the old century came to a close, however, shampooing became more common. Hairdressers in the early 1890s began offering something called *shampooing sec* (dry shampoo), which used *éther de pétrole*. This method allowed hair to dry immediately, so it did not require *séchage*, and left it very soft to the touch. On the other hand, it was a noxious and extremely volatile substance that produced more than a few accidents.[44] As indoor plumbing and water heaters worked their way through the urban landscape, *shampooing sec* fell out of favor. Coiffeurs installed *accumulateurs* and *chauffes eau instané* (*à pression* – out of a small hose) for washing hair in their salons, as hot water and soapy shampoos became the rule.[45]

Better personal hygiene improved the nation's health and, from hairdressers' perspective, made for more pleasant work. It also made a substantial contribution to their bottom line. Master coiffeur and businessman, René Rambaud, calculated that the average *française* before the war visited her coiffeur for twenty shampooings a year, at 5 francs a piece. By 1925, she indulged herself in thirty-six shampooings a year, at 8 francs per treatment.[46] For Rambaud,

43. Weber, *France*, p. 60.
44. On 'shampooing *sec*' see Spale, *Manuel*, pp. 122–3; and Rambaud, *Les fugitives*, p. 115.
45. Joyeux, 'Le gaz chez les coiffeurs.'
46. *La Coiffure de Paris*, June 1925.

the most notable thing about clean hair was its impact on hairdressers' profits. He might have added that it also reflected a remarkable turnaround in expectations and practices of popular cleanliness – a rise in the threshold of shame and disgust – made possible by technologies that brought cheap hot water to the urban masses.

The difference in sensibility and practice can be seen in the advice that experts offered women between the wars. In 1923, professors Kauffmann and Barth, of the hairdressers' training facility in Strasbourg, recommended a shampoo about once a month. They added that a light oil treatment after each shampoo would keep hair from drying out. A decade later, Georges-Lévy counseled women with long hair to wash it once every four or five weeks, those with short hair somewhat more often, and most men every other week.[47] These recommendations might fall short of contemporary habits, but they marked an enormous distance from the practices described by Antoine and Eugen Weber.

However, as Long pointed out repeatedly, the foundation of modern hairdressing was neither shampoo nor postiche nor hair coloring, but waving. The seminal moment in this respect was the invention of the 'Marcel' wave, which had burst upon coiffure in the mid 1880s and revitalized the trade. René Rambaud, probably its greatest practitioner after Marcel himself, called it 'the most important event' in the history of the profession, 'a technical, artistic, economic revolution.'[48] Marcel's *ondulation* quickly acquired a mythical quality, and many stories circulated about his epiphany. The truth goes something like this. Born in 1852, Marcel Grateau began his career inauspiciously. Finishing his apprenticeship in the provincial town of Chauvigny, Marcel came to Paris, bringing along his adored, widowed mother. For the first several years he struggled. After being fired by several employers for 'insufficient attention to cleaning up, professional incapacity,' and other misdemeanors, he installed himself in a small shop on the rue Dunkerque. During the day, according to Rambaud, Marcel coiffed 'tarts' for half a franc. At night he made wigs for the theater. A few years later Marcel bought a salon closer to the center of town, but he continued to work in anonymity until 1882, when he hit upon his 'génial' invention.[49]

The key to Marcel's technique lay in his perfection of a new type of curling

47. Kauffmann and Barth, *Le livret du coiffeur*, p. 101; Georges-Lévy, *Hygiène du cuir*, p. 12.

48. Rambaud, *Les fugitives*, p. 93.

49. For biographies of Marcel see André Bardet, *Technologie de la Coiffure* (Paris: Dervy, 1950), p. 175; Corson, *Fashions in Hair*, p. 682; d'Assailly, *Fards et Beauté*, p. 163; Gerbod, *Histoire*, p. 215; André Gissler, *Technologie de la coiffure pour dames et messieurs* (Paris:

iron – two branches, one hollow, the other round – which he used upside down, with the cylinder on top. He was thereby able to produce a wave that was soft, supple, and relatively durable. Celebrity did not arrive overnight, but one evening in 1885 Marcel had the opportunity to wave the hair of actress Jane Hading for her triumph in the play, *Le maître des forges*: 'not a single hairpin, not a single piece of false hair,' just a wave from top to bottom. Marcel's success was phenomenal. Soon *le tout Paris* wanted its hair to be waved by him and him alone. The Princesses of Sagan and von Furstenberg, the Comtesse de Castellane; actresses Réjane and Caroline Otéro; *demimondaines* Liane de Pougy, Irma de Bury, Emilienne d'Alençon – all lined up in his waiting room. His wife even considered apportioning his services by lottery. Marcel, incidentally, never actually dressed his clients' hair. He left that to others. The Master merely provided the inimitable waves.

Marcel went on to make a fortune. While most coiffeurs were able to charge between 10 and 20 francs for waving a head of hair – and this was already an important new source of income – Marcel could command 500! Thus, at a time when a coiffeur at a decent ladies salon could count on barely 500 francs a month and an assistant in a barbershop 200 francs,[50] Marcel was earning 10,000 francs a month. By 1897, according to Rambaud, having saved well over a million francs, Marcel retired to his chateau in Normandy. Marcel had little to do with the profession after his retirement, save as an icon. Besides, correspondence with him was difficult because, as Rambaud explained, 'the master was virtually illiterate.' He died in 1936.

Despite its clear popular appeal, the 'Marcel' wave initially had its opponents within the profession. Waving caused a simplification and lightening of hairstyles, and this displeased the crusty old traditionalists, whose skill lay in postiche and in the construction of elaborate (and very expensive) coiffures.[51] 'A bas l'ondulation!' was the title an 1893 article by Georges Dupuy, president of the École Française de Coiffure, as he likened the 'Marcel' to the anarchist bombs then exploding around Paris.[52]

Dunod, 1955), p. 12; Lebas and Jacques, *La coiffure*, pp. 253–4; and René Rambaud, *L'onduation bouclée. Trois méthodes d'ondulation en une seule* (Paris: Société d'Editions Modernes Parisiennes, 1949), pp. 46–7.

50. Desplanques, *Barbiers*, p. 215.

51. Theodore Zeldin (*France*, p. 441.) gave the following prices for *hautes coiffures* of the 1880s:
  – 5 francs for an ordinary styling
  – 15–20 for a powdered coiffure
  – 20–30 for a 'historic' style
  – 30–40 for a coiffure for a costume ball ('coiffure du genre pour transvestissement').

52. Gerbod, *Histoire*, p. 193; Rambaud, *Les fugitives*, pp. 109–10.

Such criticism, however, could not sway a determined public opinion, and waving quickly became the essential element in virtually all hairstyles. The 'Marcel' ruled coiffure 'de manière quasi absolue' until after World War I, bringing expansion and prosperity to the profession. Eventually, even Dupuy recanted: 'Vive la Marcel,' he wrote in 1907. It was generally thought that none of his emulators was able to match the softness and beauty of Marcel's waves, and the Master kept his secrets to himself. Nonetheless, if the details of his method remained obscure, the general principles were widely known. Ondulation was soon the most important skill learned by young *coiffeurs* and *coiffeuses pour dames*. Indeed, Long noted ruefully, it was often their only skill. Semi-skilled labor, in effect, was replacing art.

By the end of the Belle Epoque barely a head was dressed that did not include some waving. Its popularity extended to all segments of the population, from the most fashionable *bourgeoises* to factory girls and shop assistants. Long reacted with typical ambivalence to the democratization of the 'Marcel.' He applauded the fact that increasing numbers of women from all classes were beginning to visit *salons de coiffure*, paying up to 10 or 20 francs on each occasion. On the other hand, he remained uncomfortable with the decline in quality that accompanied waving down the social ladder. He noted in 1918 that while the *ondulations* produced in elegant shops were large, soft, and delicate, 'with the lower grade of customer frequenting the cheaper class of establishment, one sees curls that are too frizzy and waves which are much too pronounced' – waves that, as Antoine put it, resembled 'the general lines of the rougher part of a wash-board.'[53]

Fine and soft or cheap and frizzy, all *ondulations* shared the same shortcoming. At the end of a humid evening or after a couple of weeks, even the most exquisitely waved hair would return to its natural state. Long was naturally intrigued, therefore, by a new invention attracting attention on the other side of the English Channel. In 1906, in London, a German-born hairdresser by the name of Charles Nestlé gave the first demonstration of his wondrous, if somewhat terrifying, apparatus – a machine to give hair a wave that would last for six months, through rain, humidity, and shampooing.[54]

The technique for *frisure forcée* was an old recipe of the *posticheur's* trade. Hair was divided into locks (*mèches*), soaked in alkaline solution, and boiled.

---

53. Graves, *Devotion*, p. 37.

54. On the permanent wave see *La Coiffure de Paris*, October 1920; Lebas and Jacques, *La Coiffure*, p. 308–10; Volo Litvinsky, *Toute la permanente. Tous les procédés et tours de mains* (Paris: Société d'Editions Modernes Parisiennes, 1949), pp. 13–15; Rambaud, *Les fugitives*, pp. 167–70; Spale, *Manuel*, pp. 234–9.

For obvious reasons, this process was impractical for hair still attached to the client. Nestlé's breakthrough was inventing a machine that could boil a woman's hair without scalding her scalp, more or less. He rolled the locks into curlers (*bigoudis*) – thirty or fifty would cover a head – which were then wrapped and subjected to heat from an electric current. The hair could then be washed out and dressed.

Long saw the potential of *frisure forcée*, and in 1907 he brought Nestlé and his contraption to Paris for a demonstration. Long's colleagues, it was reported, remained unimpressed with the result – and apparently with some reason. Nestlé's machine, though ingenious, was crude. It required four to five hours to complete the process and produced waves that, in the words of René Rambaud, had a 'truly repulsive look' to them. Nevertheless, Nestlé had surmounted an important technological barrier and he was quickly followed by others who improved on his method. In 1918, Eugene Sutter, also in England, brought out a machine that, according to Long, made the permanent wave process easier, simpler, and more certain, eliminating 'the risk of curling like a poodle dog a head of hair which required only a few large and soft waves.'[55] A year later, Gaston Boudou introduced the first French-made machine, the 'Gallia,' followed shortly by the 'Perma Standard,' the 'Wella,' and a host of others.

The permanent wave appealed to women's increasing demand for convenience, along with their desire to be youthful, sporty, and fashionable. A 1920 advertisement in *Vogue* magazine promised:

All hairstyles are possible with the permanent-wave system, Emile [Gallia], the most advanced system, giving absolutely permanent waves. After a bath, an automobile outing, a game of tennis or golf, under a rainstorm, after a foxtrot, your coiffure will be more becoming, thanks to the resistance of the *ondulations*, while those limp locks of hair, which ordinarily look so sadly neglected, once they are waved, will add charm and lightness to any hairstyle.[56]

By Long's account, French hairdressers were initially skeptical about the *machine à l'indéfrisable*, as the permanent wave machines came to be called, but their reticence soon gave way before their recognition of the indéfrisable's unprecedented commercial possibilities, as the taste for permanent waves spread through the population. Consider the figures. The average cost of a treatment in the *fauteuil* and under the machine *à l'indéfrisable* was 10 francs per *mèche*, or 300 to 500 francs for an entire head. The waving itself had to

55. *HWJS*, March 1919.
56. *Vogue*, 1 December 1920, p. vi.

be followed by setting and dressing, and a conscientiously groomed woman would return weekly to have her wave refreshed and twice a year for a full 'perm.' The permanent wave turned out to be an undeniable bonanza for the hairdressing profession.

It proved particularly suitable for the shorter styles that came into fashion after the war. Rambaud wrote that the *indéfrisable* allowed even *cheveux courts* to remain stylish and feminine, and meant that a woman could be 'bien coiffée' with just a few strokes of her hairbrush. It is quite possible, he concluded, that short hairstyles would never have attained their fantastic popularity without permanent waves.[57]

This amounted to an impressive claim for the *indéfrisable*, because no fashion trend of the first quarter of the century could match the profound impact of the vogue for women's short hair that swept, not only through France, but across Western civilization. In its popularity and its radical departure from the voluminous styles that preceded it, the 'bob,' as it was generally known, looked like evidence of a revolution in society and popular consciousness. By the mid-1920s, there seemed hardly a woman who had not cut her hair 'à la garçonne' (in a 'boyish look'). Rich and poor, *jeune fille* and *grande mère*, all of them joined in the interring of old standards of womanhood.

At least that is how it appeared to those who watched in horror as one of the most powerful symbols of femininity tumbled onto salon floors. Some coiffeurs feared *cheveux courts* because their "art" required long hair. Most worried about its effect on business; without long tresses to be weaved, waved, and adorned, would women have any further use for their coiffeurs? For religious authorities, natality experts, and social conservatives in general, women with short hair represented something entirely more sinister: a 'civilization without sexes,' the end of France.[58] Even within families, scandal

---

57. Rambaud, who began as Boudou's protégé and worked closely with him, became a corporate spokesman for the Gallia company and wrote a monthly column for its journal, *Gallia*. See especially March–April 1926 for Rambaud's reflections on the relationship of the 'perm' to ladies' short hairstyles.

58. The phrase 'civilization without sexes' comes from the pen of the fascist writer, Pierre Drieu la Rochelle, and I borrow it from Roberts, *Civilization Without Sexes*. There is a huge literature on the phenonemon of the 'Garçonne,' the name drawn from the novel by Victor Margueritte. Roberts' bibliography is comprehensive, but see also Steven Zdatny, 'La mode à la garçonne, 1900–1925: une histoire sociale des coupes de cheveux,' *Le Mouvement Social* 174 (January–March 1996), pp. 23–56; Anne-Marie Sohn, 'Between the Wars in England and France,' and Françoise Thébaud, 'The Great War and the Triumph of Sexual Division,' both in Thébaud, ed., *A History of Women in the West, Vol. V: Toward a Cultural identity in the Twentieth Century* (Cambridge MA: Harvard U. Press, 1994).

and violence accompanied the action of scissors and clippers, as outraged husbands and fathers reacted angrily to this perceived challenge to their authority. Rambaud told the story of a father who sued a coiffeur for cutting his daughter's hair without his authorization. Such outrage was common.[59]

The notoriety attaching to the 'bob' led many to claim authorship. In one frequently repeated story, Antoine took credit for having invented the 'coupe à la Jeanne d'Arc' when, in 1909, he cropped the hair of Eve Lavallière, in order to fit the forty-year-old actress to the part of the eighteen-year-old heroine of *L'Ane de Buridan*. Sometimes a different yarn was spun – of the young Gabrielle 'Coco' Chanel – although the critical moment for her arrived a few years later. It seems that one evening in 1917, when Chanel was still devoted primarily to designing hats, she was getting ready to attend the opera when her gas heater exploded near her head, leaving her hair singed and smoky. Coco first thought to cancel her *soirée*. Then, with the audacity for which she soon became famous, she took nail scissors and cut off her braids. Appearing at the opera with short hair and a hip-waisted, short dress, Chanel caused a sensation. The next day, so the legend goes, Misia Edwards, Mme Letellier, and Celia Sorel, who had seen her the previous evening, all went to Chanel to have their own hair cut with the now-celebrated nail scissors.[60] Yet another myth attributed the inspiration for *cheveux courts* to the American nurses, who brought it with them to France during the war.[61]

The truth of the matter is that short hairstyles captured the public's fancy in a more gradual and anonymous manner, in the same way that the Edwardian ideal of feminine perfection eventually ceded to the 'flapper.' In 1908, the 'modernist' couturier, Paul Poiret, had broken dramatically with convention when he chopped the models' hair for that year's collection. The dancers Irene Castle and Isadora Duncan, and the actress Iris Storm, were already sporting 'bobs' well before the First World War.[62] Without a doubt, its adoption by the young lionesses of Paris Society, and especially the publicity it received from the likes of Antoine and Chanel, helped to propel the 'bob' to fashion prominence, but *cheveux courts* had no single author, as such.

Long first mentioned short hairstyles in August 1910. He did not like them. 'Today we should consider it a crime of lèse beauty to pass the scissors over

---

59. See especially Anne Manson, 'La scandale de "la garçonne,"' in Gilbert Guilleminault, ed., *Les années folles* (Paris: Denoël, 1958), p. 153; and Rambaud, *Les fugitives*, pp. 240–41.

60. See Galant, *Les années Chanel*, p. 68; Haedrich, *Coco Chanel*, p. 149.

61. D'Assailly, *Fards et beauté*, p. 163; Corson, *Fashions in Hair*, p. 613; *Gallia Journal*, March–April 1926; Rambaud, *Les fugitives*, p. 195.

62. Ecksteins, *Rites of Spring*, p. 259; and Valerie Steele, *Paris Fashion: A Cultural History* (New York: Oxford U. Press, 1988), p. 246.

a healthy head of hair,' he wrote. It was not until 1917, in fact, that Long began to pay the 'bob' any serious attention. In May of that year, he observed that the 'smart set' were cutting their hair, although even so-called short styles remained a foot long and eminently dressable. As for more radical cuts like the 'Jeanne d'Arc,' Long expressed confidence that 'modern women are not at all stupid enough to adopt such a style.' Only as the war was coming to an end and the daily newspapers were filled with discussions of the striking vogue for short hairstyles, did Long gradually begin to accept them. As late as February 1919, when the 'bob' was attaining epidemic proportions, Long was still campaigning against 'this freakish whim' that made 'women, with their overdone make-up and peculiar head-dresses, look more like clowns straight from the circus than any category of female.'

The following May, while consoling himself that short hairstyles were only 'a passing fashion, and one which is already beginning to pass,' Long speculated on the genesis of this unpleasant mode. Short hair, he wrote, was a sign of the times: 'The woman who works becomes manly . . . Feminism is rising [and] is not woman's long hair a sign of servitude? Short hair typifies a programme of franchise, as we are given to understand, when a wise woman orders her hair to be cut and dresses *à l'indépendance*.' The 'bob' was also a response to historic tumult. Just as 'short coiffures appeared after the *Terreur* [of the French Revolution], Notre Dame de Thermidor[63] had short hair, and the beautiful ladies who escaped the guillotine wore their hair "à la victime,"' wrote Long, the present fashion of *cheveux courts* derived from the trauma of the war and the Russian Revolution.

Long's disdain for them was but a pale reflection of the ferocious attacks directed at short hairstyles by conservatives frightened by the 'New Woman.' After all, Long's primary interest in short hair was not political; it was aesthetic and commercial. He treated the 'bob' as just another hairstyle, of interest to coiffeurs for its charm (or lack of it) and its profitability, and not because it betokened decadence and the imminent end of civilization. If he disliked *cheveux courts*, it was because he thought them ugly and feared they would cost hairdressers money. In any case, by 1920 Long's fears on this account had dispersed because he, along with his colleagues, discovered that even short hair could be filled with ornaments and waves. The 'New Woman,' whatever her deep symbolic significance, was turning out to be profitable for hairdressers.

The dimensions of coiffure's rising fortunes are easy enough to discern. The total number of people employed as hairdressers rose from under 48,000

63. Zdatny, 'La mode à la garçonne,' pp. 44–5.

in 1896 to almost 62,000 in 1926 and to over 125,000 by 1936. Note that these global figures understate the particular explosion in *coiffure pour dames*, because the number of barbers was itself diminishing. It was universally conceded that the profession was becoming both larger and more prosperous, at least until the late 1920s.

Moreover, it was not merely as customers that women were acquiring a more prominent role in coiffure. More and more of them were entering the profession as workers and shop owners. The proportion of women in the profession grew remarkably, from 10.2 per cent in the 1896 census to 36.5 per cent in 1936. In Paris the process was even more dramatic, as *coiffeuses* increased from 8.5 per cent of the working population in coiffure in 1896 to 43.5 per cent (and 45 percent of salon owners) 40 years later.[64]

Once more, the war accelerated a trend that had begun in the Belle Epoque. With so many men gone off to the front, women increasingly took their places in the salons. Wives ran their departed husbands' businesses; daughters flocked to the *écoles de coiffure*, which were glad to have the students. Indeed, the war opened a window of substantial opportunity for *coiffeuses*. We can see this most clearly in Long's article of July 1917, which he devoted to the 'female ladies' hairdressers of Paris.' He recorded their youth and eagerness, the good work they were doing, and especially the chance they were enjoying to earn good money. 'There are many girls with their hair still in plaits and not yet 15,' he wrote, 'who earn from 6 to 8 francs per day . . . Wavers who are a little older obtain about double.'

If Long did not use his reports to his English colleagues to fulminate against the end of *la différance* and the violation of ideal womanhood, he nonetheless had some very strong notions of what a woman should be and, indeed, of what she *naturally* was. How could it have been otherwise for a man whose life was dedicated to satisfying women's most supercilious desires?

Thus we read in Long's articles frequent allusions to women's innate and irrepressible 'regard for coquetry,' flowing from those laws of nature that intended women to have pretty hair. 'The more civilized and cultured a woman becomes,' Long wrote in May 1913, 'the more she resembles the savage of the Pacific Islands in her taste for showy colors and glittering ornaments.' Similar preconceptions about 'eternal' femininity pervaded the fashion – that is, the coquetry – business, just as they permeated the rest of society, where women's supposed attachment to life's shallower concerns was taken for evidence of their inferiority.[65]

64. For a good discussion of the period's misogyny see Roberts, *Civilization Without Sexes*, passim.

65. A reference to the revolutionary month (27 July 1794) in which Robespierre was overthrown and the Terror ended.

Long believed that Nature reached its apotheosis in the fashionable ladies on 'holiday' in one of the seaside resorts – 'slaves of their existence . . . for fifteen hours a day'[66] and yet, at that very moment, just beyond Long's view, stylish *young* women in short hair and lighter clothing, impatient with its heavy burdens, were abandoning the more onerous rituals of a fashionably-led life.[67]

The First World War delivered a great shock to all the gendered certainties of the prewar world, and we have already seen some of its reverberations in the hairdressing profession. The war deprived women of male companionship and supervision, as husbands, sons, and fathers went off to fight. It further produced profound changes in women's economic and social circumstances. Most famously, it drew unprecedented numbers of women, even from the middle classes, into the labor market and allowed them into jobs they could never before have held.[68] Female bus conductors and munitions workers are images as central to the war experience as trenches and gas masks. Industrial work, decent wages, and a certain distance from patriarchy also brought women a new measure of autonomy and, according to some observers, self-confidence.[69]

Debate continues as to whether all this really constituted some important dose of emancipation for women and whether the consequent 'crisis of femininity' brought France to the edge of cultural collapse.[70] Long himself

66. *HWJS*, September 1920.

67. Mulvagh, *Vogue's History*, p. 45.

68. On the War's economic impact on women see Marilyn Boxer and Jean Quaetart, eds., *Connecting Spheres: Women in the Western World, 1500 to the Present* (New York: Oxford U. Press, 1987), pp. 193–5 and 208; Yvonne Delatour, 'Le travail des femmes pendant la première guerre mondiale et ses conséqences sur l'évolution de leur rôle dans la société,' *Francia* 2 (1974), pp. 1482–501; Laura Lee Downs, *Manufacturing Inequality: Gender Division in the French and British Metalworking Industries, 1914–1939* (Ithaca: Cornell U. Press, 1995); Françoise Thébaud, *La femme au temps de la guerre de 14* (Paris: Stock, 1986), pp. 158–67; and idem, 'The Great War and the Triumph of Sexual Division,' in Thébuad, *A History of Women*, pp. 29–34; Louise A. Tilly and Joan W. Scott, *Women, Work and Family* (New York: Holt, Rinehart & Winston, 1978).

69. On the war's social and cultural impact on women see Gabriel Perreux, *La vie quotidienne des civils en France pendant la grande guerre* (Paris: Hachette, 1966), pp. 63–7; Mary Louise Roberts, 'This Civilization No Longer Has Sexes: La Garçonne and the Cultural Crisis in France After World War I,' *Gender and History* 4:1 (Spring 1992), pp. 49–69; idem, *Civilization Without Sexes*, p. 6; and Thébaud, 'The Great War,' passim. For England see Arthur Marwick, *The Deluge: British Society and the First World War* (New York: Norton, 1965), and idem, *Women at War, 1914–1918* (London: Fontana, 1977).

70. For some 'pop' analyses of the war's liberating effect see Antoine, *J'ai coiffé*, p. 110; Charles-Roux, *L'irrégulière*, p. 226; Rambaud, *Les fugitives*, p. 203; Rambaud, *Les qualités nécessaires à un coiffeur pour dames. Physiques, morales, psychologiques, techniques et*

evinced little interest in these Big Questions, yet his articles from the war years read like a serial essay on the war's impact on fashion and social life. The pieces he wrote in the early summer of 1914 described a profession enjoying a moment of prosperity. The turban craze, which had so badly hurt the waving business, was but a faint memory. The 'Marcel' wave was back in vogue and being liberally incorporated into high, ornate coiffures that kept ladies' hairdressers busy and financially content.

This air of optimism quickly dissipated with the outbreak of war, which dealt the peripheral industries of fashion and leisure a sharp blow. Restaurants, theaters, and racetracks closed. Conspicuous consumption, where it was not prohibited outright by the military government, was suppressed by public sensibilities.[71] Virtually the whole peacetime economy was suspended while the country geared up for a short, intense conflict.[72] As life on the home front was reduced to its essentials, those who made a living by the inessentials faced bleak prospects.

Under the circumstances, Long posed the obvious question: how could hairdressers survive the collapse of their customary business? The answers he proposed were ingenious, but their very ingenuity pointed to the desperate state of affairs. In his articles of September and October 1914, 'Hairdressing for Girls,' Long advised his readers to cultivate the potential market in 'infants and juveniles' and apply themselves to such mundane tasks as shampooing and dressing very plain coiffures. In the months that followed, he offered instructions on the making of dolls' wigs and the manufacture of 'bracelets, chains, rings,' and other ghastly mementos for departing loved ones made from human hair.

Even where fashion survived, the war brought an end to flamboyance. Long, perhaps putting the best face on a bad situation, first applauded the simplification of hairstyles:

The effect of the war will be to banish the excessive exaggerations of Fashion that were approaching almost to folly. What extravagance of shape and proportions,

---

artistiques. Conférence faite le 24 novembre 1933 à l'Ecole de Coiffure de Paris (pamphlet, 1933). For a skeptical view of the matter see Steven C. Hause, 'More Minerva than Mars: The French Women's Rights Campaign and the First World War,' in Margaret R. Higonnet, Jane Jenson, Sonya Michel and Margaret Collins Weitz, eds., *Between the Lines: Gender and the Two World Wars* (New Haven: Yale U. Press, 1987).

71. On the disruption of amusement and consumption see Mulvagh, *Vogue's History*, p.11; Rambaud, *Les fugitives*, p.188; Rearick, *Pleasures of the Belle Epoque*, p. 214; and Wiser, *Crazy Years*, p. 73.

72. See Jean-Jacques Becker, *The Great War and the French People* (Leamington Spa: Berg, 1985), especially 'Part I Autumn 1914,' pp. 9–102.

for instance, the feminine headdress had attained when the war suddenly brought us back to more moderate and wiser sentiments and more modest tastes.

Yet in the next breath he warned against 'exaggerations . . . in simplicity' that resembled neglect and that ran counter to women's natural inclination to 'look after [their] hair.'[73]

It turned out that Long had worried needlessly about the suppression of women's natural tendencies. For even as he wrote, the fashion instinct was beginning to reassert itself. As early as July 1915, Long reported the reopening of a 'first-class restaurant' in Paris, catering to the rich, who were reviving Paris Society – on behalf, it was said, of war charities. In fact, while they continued from time to time to lament the enforced simplicity of wartime fashions, Long's essays from the middle of 1915 onwards testify to a 'normal-ization' of fashion life.[74] He no longer wrote about morbid keepsakes and children's hair but returned to familiar themes of hairstyles and profits. In February 1916, the first shells fired at Verdun coincided with the return of the highly elaborate '1830 style of dress.' As the battle drew to a bloody close nine months later, Long described the young women of Paris wearing 'coiffures extremely high, skirts excessively short, dresses decidedly *décolleté*, and faces inordinately painted.' As the British launched their attack on Passchendaele Ridge in September 1917, Long reported that the *maisons* of Paris were closed, because *la haute société* was still off at the summer resorts. Long's interest in the war itself faded to the occasional platitude.

Extravagance in the middle of the war obviously struck many people as inappropriate, and it produced a backlash. A public controversy ensued over the lavishness of the 'feminine toilet' and the propriety of 'dressing up' and 'going out' at a moment of such profound tragedy. In January 1917, Long mentioned a recent ban on the wearing of evening dress to the theater. He considered this puritanism misguided. Weighing the interests of propriety against those of commerce, Long declared himself for the latter, so as not to deprive 'thousands of workers of their means of livelihood.' 'No matter how grave the situation may be,' he argued, 'one ought never to prevent persons who have the money from spending it, and even generously.' Besides, the suppression of fashion would work a particular hardship on women if their 'innate regard for coquetry remains unsatisfied.'[75]

As long as the war lasted, the tension between propriety and extravagance was never resolved. Long's articles made it clear that whereas almost everyone

73. *HWJS*, September 1915.
74. Also see Perreux, *La vie quotidienne*, pp. 262–3.
75. *HWJS*, November 1916 and February 1917.

acknowledged the need for restraint, many women from across the social spectrum continued to apply themselves to being stylish – even if in a more subdued manner. The end of the war, however, released the fashionable classes from whatever inhibitions had constrained them. The celebratory galas and 'victory balls' that followed the Armistice carried caprice to new heights. Long described what he called the 'Restoration mentality' that he likened the post-Robespierre days of the *Merveilleuses*, extravagant and *déshabillées*: 'Ladies reveal their shoulders; corsets have, so to speak, disappeared; and the habit of applying a depilatory beneath the arms has been acquired.' Hairstyles were short, skirts shorter, stockings sheer or even absent, legs made clean by the safety razors now in every lady's toilette cabinet – and this 'in spite of the unheard-of prices of everything.'[76]

The styles affected by those young women who danced and flirted their nights away at the victory galas differed dramatically from those that had reigned before the war. The Edwardian woman, enclosed in corset and bustle – designer Paul Poiret wrote that he 'waged war' upon this style that 'divided its wearer into two distinct masses' and made her look' as if she were hauling a trailer'[77] – could hardly have cut a more dissimilar figure from the young flapper with bobbed hair and Chanel jersey. It was impossible not to notice the change that had occurred, and the most common explanation was that the war was directly responsible for it. It seemed obvious and logical that simpler, freer styles, needing less material and allowing easier movement, were a product of the war's demands for women's austerity and work, just as the autonomy they had acquired in men's absence made them more assertive. It was widely thought that, as the war had liberated women in a general way, it had also led them to demand less confining and more convenient fashions – a process that designers could not then reverse.[78]

Others, especially in retrospect, have recognized the radical transformation of styles but doubted that fashions so faithfully reflected historical circumstances.[79] After all, there was nothing unprecedented in the straight lines of Chanel designs or in the short haircuts of the 'garçonnes.' It was merely the

---

76. *HWJS*, July 1919 and December 1919.

77. Poiret, *King of Fashion*, p. 76.

78. See, for example, Antoine, *J'ai coiffé*, p. 110; Charles-Roux, *L'irrégulière*, p. 226; Rambaud, *Les fugitives*, pp. 195–96.

79. Styles had changed, wrote James McMillan in *Housewife or Harlot: The Place of Women in French Society, 1870–1940* (New York: St. Martin's Press, 1981), p.163, and contemporaries 'took [them] to be only the external manifestation of more profound changes.' Also see Anne-Marie Sohn, 'La garçonne face à l'opinion publique: type littéraire ou type social des années 20,' *Le Mouvement Social* (July–September 1972), p. 3.

case that what had been the cutting edge of fashion in 1914 had become the mainstream in 1920.[80] Women's fashions, wrote historian Valerie Steele, evolved gradually, according to some internal logic of the eye and the mind, and not, as is commonly proposed, to fit the need for functional dress and sexual liberation.[81] Anne Hollander agrees. 'It is not enough,' she wrote, 'to say that women adopted short skirts after the First World War because they symbolized sexual freedom and permitted easy movement of the legs, since these practical and symbolic effects could have been accomplished in other ways.' Besides, the new clothes did not really serve utility or sportiness very well – high heels, for instance, or sheer hose, or merely 'the psychologically taxing problems of looking comfortable and dressing simply while being rather exposed.'[82]

Both Steele and Hollander recognize, however, that the flapper was a phenomenon. More than just another stop in the fashion cycle, the *garçonne* signaled a decisive transition in the ideal of feminine beauty and sexuality. Where maturity had once defined the perfect woman, the emphasis was now on youthfulness.[83] The real queens of the victory balls, Long reported, were the 'young and modern ladies of elegance whom the men of wealth dote over' – for instance, a certain Mademoiselle Diamant, whom he called 'the greatest vedette of [1920].'[84]

Yet even before the war Long had begun to pay less attention to Society's *grandes dames* and to focus increasingly on the escapades of its young coquettes – of whom he wrote in March 1913 that they 'do not hesitate to wear their skirts so short as to exhibit half the length of their legs and a considerable portion of their stockings of golden lace, [but] who are very careful to hide three quarters of their faces, which are elaborately made up.'

The passion for youthfulness had consequences of both an aesthetic and commercial nature. Postwar fashion emphasized the qualities of youth: slimness, athleticism, breeziness, rebelliousness. The glorification of youth was written all over women's bodies, from short hair 'in the style of a sophisticated schoolgirl' to clothing that minimized 'matronly' breasts, while

80. Another instance of the 'outsider as insider': see Peter Gay, *Weimar Culture: The Outsider as Insider* (New York: Harper, 1968).

81. Valerie Steele, *Fashion and Eroticism: Ideals of Feminine Beauty from the Victorian Era to the Jazz Age* (New York: Oxford U. Press, 1985), p. 235; and idem, *Paris Fashion*, pp. 232–3.

82. Anne Hollander, *Seeing Through Clothes* (New York: Viking, 1975), pp. 313, 335, 339.

83. Bonnie Smith, *Changing Lives: Women in European History Since 1700* (Lexington MA: DC Heath & Co., 1989), pp. 317–26 and 410–11; Mulvagh, *Vogue's History*, pp. 10–11.

84. *HWJS*, January 1919 and October 1920.

it focused attention on 'long . . . straight . . . shapely,' and nubile legs. 'An active looking body,' noted Anne Hollander, 'became requisite for elegance.'[85] In this respect, Long's articles illuminate a social revolution. The 'bob' became the signpost that marked out a new consumer society, driven by the tastes and spending habits of young people, and especially of young women.[86]

Beyond the 'youthification' of consumption, the new consumer society was also distinguished by the expansion of the market for fashionable products across its traditional class barriers. The first tremors of this cultural earthquake were already detectable in the Belle Epoque. Long's inaugural contribution to the *Hairdressers' Weekly Journal* informed his readers that the 'Coque Normande' coiffure had spread to 'all the work girls . . . of Paris,' as the popular classes searched for distinction. And once again, the war, which did not give birth to this consumer revolution, nonetheless helped bring it to maturity. 'Parisian work girls and female employees generally,' Long wrote in November 1918, 'have now all acquired the habit of attending the hair dressers, and nearly all for waving. The cheap *salons d'ondulation* have large and increasing connections, and are open until as late as nine o'clock at night in the popular quarters.' It was becoming hard, he sighed, to distinguish 'the lady of fashion [from] her humble sister.'[87] Hair, like fashion generally, was an integral part of a developing mass culture.

Typically, the democratization of the market for coiffure both pleased Long and horrified him. On the one hand, as a businessman he could only be thrilled at the vast opportunities opening up for hairdressers as the hoi polloi flocked to their local beauty salons. On the other, Long, who was at bottom a terrible snob, was appalled at what often emerged. 'The waving that is done in these [cheap] establishments,' he grumbled, 'has a special character of its own, which can be recognised from afar – a sort of rigid, set, regular groove, very pronounced and so formal that it can be compared to the effect seen in woodcarving.'[88] He did not mean it as a compliment.

Indeed, nothing testified to the democratization of *ondulation* more than the efforts of the swell set to leave it behind. At postwar celebrations, amidst the 'diamond bands, materials of gold, magnificent feathers and combs . . .

---

85. Steele, *Fashion and Eroticism*, p. 239; Hollander, *Seeing Through Clothes*, p. 338.
86. René Koenig, 'La diffusion de la mode dans les sociétés contemporaines,' *Cahiers Internationaux de Sociologie* 63 (July–December 1961), p. 40; idem, *Sociologie de la mode* (Paris: Petite Bibliothèque Payot, 1969). On the youthification and feminization of mass consumption see also Kathy Peiss, *Cheap Amusements: Working Women and Leisure in Turn-of-the-Century New York* (Philadelphia: Temple U. Press, 1986); and Peiss, 'Commercial Leisure and the "Woman Question,"' in Butsch, *For Fun and Profit*, pp. 102–17.
87. *HWJS*, March 1917.
88. *HWJS*, November 1918.

to be seen everywhere,' Long observed that the chic new coiffures employed hardly any wave. This, he noted, 'pleases not a little those ladies who wish to be different from the factory girls and their "well-marked" shilling waving.'[89]

Taken together, Emile Long's reports on Paris coiffure offer the reader a casual and idiosyncratic chronicle of a critical period, stretching from the Belle Epoque, through the Great War, to the doorstep of the 'roaring twenties'. In narrow focus, Long provides an archive of fashion, an ongoing catalogue of coiffures, hat styles, and clothing design – amply illustrated with pen and anecdote. Were waves in or out? Did ladies wear their chignons high or low? What were the most beautiful and profitable additions to the latest coiffure? What were the *couturiers* and milliners planning for the coming season, and what would that mean for hairdressers? Long aimed simply to enhance feminine beauty and coiffeurs' revenues, not to keep a journal of social change.

However, if we lengthen the focus, we find that Long describes a social and cultural revolution. The expansion of *coiffure pour dames*, the increasing use of hair color and the *machine à l'indéfrisable*, and perhaps most of all, the irrepressible taste for *cheveux courts* were all reflections of profound changes in French society. For the evolution of the hairdressing profession was propelled by the increasing participation of working- and lower-middle class women in the economy of fashion, and by the disproportionate impact of *young* women on this process. Long illustrates the fact that these forces were already in motion before the war, but that the war hastened their progress, so that what had been the vague outlines of the future in 1914 were distinctly and powerfully clear in 1919. Between 1910 and 1920, Long's commentaries transport us from the consumer society of the nineteenth century into that of the twentieth.

A coiffure, it turns out, may be in itself a frivolous thing, yet it is anchored in the structures and mentalities that define a society. In its composition and commercial disposition we can discern technological growth, class relations, the reconstruction of gender, the birth of mass consumerism. That, in the end, is the value of Long's essays: a series of reports on hair and fashion, they can be read as the history of an age.

89. *HWJS*, July 1919.

1

January 7, 1910: Decline of the Turban Headdress in Paris

[*Occupying through his many Trade and literary connections a unique position for the acquirement of early and authentic information, our Paris correspondent supplies details in the following article of what the fashion in hairdressing is likely to be during the coming Spring. He also contributes an interesting survey of the events and causes which eventuated in the 'turban craze,' which, however, he says, is fast subsiding in the best circles of the French capital.*]

It will, I imagine, be generally conceded that Marcel waving constitutes for the ladies' hairdresser a great Trade improvement – an excellent means of enhancing the appearance of the human hair and of the feminine headdress. From the point of view of the public, Marcel waving is indisputably an important element in the ladies' toilet. Consequently, it will not – it *cannot* – disappear. But its great popularity, which was described, and not without reason, as bordering almost on a craze, undoubtedly diminished during the year 1909. We who have followed its history know how tenacious has been its hold, how remunerative it has been to the Trade, and what truly artistic headdresses it has made possible during its long reign.

Having recounted at length how this unprecedented demand originated,[1] I may now appropriately relate the reasons for its almost equally sudden decline. The Circumstances form quite an interesting story.

The Decline of Marcel Waving

We have in Paris an important daily newspaper, the proprietor of which, M. Pierre Letellier, is very rich. He married a young lady of rare beauty. Mme. Letellier, in fact, has the reputation of being the handsomest woman in Paris. She is also one of the most elegant, for she possesses splendid taste as well as ample means. Consequently, she is much sought after, much talked about, and to a large extent imitated; that is to say, in common with one or two

---

1. In Emile Long, *Traité complet et illustré de l'ondulation*, serialized as 'A Complete Treatise on Hair Waving,' in the *Hairdressers' Weekly Journal Supplement*.

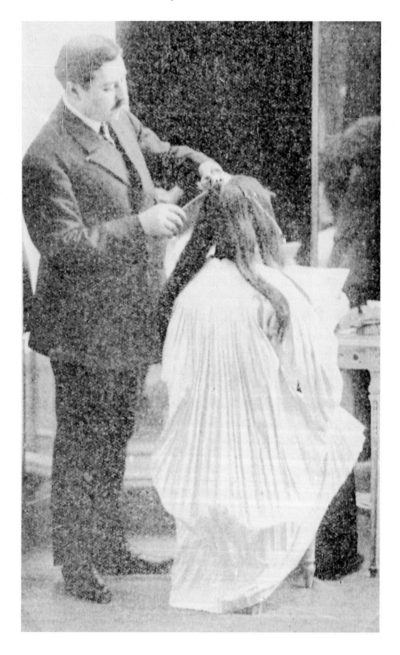

Figure 1. 'Emile Long – Les Divisions': The master combs his client's hair into *mèches* before waving it. From Emile Long, *L'attrape-science de la coiffure féminine, avec seize photos* (Paris: Encyclopédie Professionnelle du 'Capilartiste', 1912).

young and popular actresses, she is the subject of a general public curiosity and admiration, and what she adopts for her toilet and for her headdresses are accepted as the proper styles of the moment.

Whilst the hair of Mme. Letellier was waved nobody would have dreamed of suppressing one single effect of the [curling] iron. There came a day, however (it was at Trouville,[2] during the summer season), when painters and artists belonging to the modern school found Mme. Letellier so beautiful, so seductive – so rich, also, perhaps – that they resolved to commit her beauty, her graceful, harmonious elegance, to canvas. It is known that these modern artists have a horror for waving; being lacking in the patience of the Old Masters, they cannot easily depict the alternating lights and shades of Marcel's invention, and so they grasp at any means of extricating themselves from the difficulties of the situation.

Thus we find that the young painter La Gandara proceeded to remodel Mme. Letellier's headdress entirely before painting her portrait, and although, as I know, he devised a very tasty coiffure, it departed altogether from the prevailing fashion.

Then came the artist Helleu, who was soon a friend of the family, and whom M. Letellier rendered famous in less than a year because of the great publicity he gave to him in his newspaper. Whilst Helleu did not re-model Mme. Letellier's coiffure, he evinced no inclination to depict its undulations. During the year 1908 he produced quite a number of portraits in pencil, in which her features were well portrayed, but her hair was always absolutely straight, contrary to the style actually adopted by the beautiful model.

Soon M. Helleu was famous. All the young women of the modernist school were anxious to have their portraits done by him, and the artist represented them all with beautiful eyes and straight hair!

Afterwards, the lady artists attached to *Femina* [a fashion magazine] (and particularly the one who signs herself 'Driant') imitated the example of Helleu; the details of the elegant gowns they represented were faithfully reproduced as hitherto, but the coiffures were disposed of with a few strokes of the pencil; and that is how the impression came about – first in the upper select circle and later amongst the great public – that it was not necessary to wave so much – that, in fact, waving was no longer the fashion.

The Advent of the Turban Headdress

This was at the commencement of the year 1909. The models designed to display the new gowns in the important journal *Femina* were all drawn with straight hair, in direct and striking contrast to the illustrations of hairdressing

2. The trendy resort in Normandy, on the English Channel.

published in the same paper by the hairdressers who advertised in it. The latter, agitated at the turn of affairs, sent to the editor a collective protest, penned by our colleague, M. Heng, to the effect that they would withdraw all their advertisements if the artists attached to the paper continued, through their drawings, to prejudice the interests of the Hairdressing Trade. The editor was a little surprised and embarrassed, but he apologised very politely and promised to give orders that the grievances should be redressed.

But did he do it? In any case, it was already too late. The harm had been done, for the Journal *de luxe* [i.e., *Femina*], in spite of its high price, circulates more than 150,000 copies each fortnight, and goes into every corner of the world.

The ladies' hairdressers, intoxicated for a long time by their easy success, had neglected to group themselves together in readiness to deal with such an eventuality, and so they were helpless to counteract the seriousness of the position. Every day clients would call on them with pages torn from the great *Femina*, and request that their hair should be dressed according to the latest fashion – they did not want waving, or waved postiche, any longer. Harassed by customers on the one hand, and by the public Press on the other, the hairdressers laid aside their irons reluctantly, and to meet the requirements of the 'cocoa-nut' coiffure, sought from the bottom of their drawers all the long hair that they possessed, in order to produce postiche in keeping with the new style. Turbans were hastily resuscitated under the name of '*calot*,' and the old wide, flat chignon, which the peasants of Brittany and Normandy still wear, and which enjoyed celebrity formerly in Paris under the name of '*Coque Normande*,' was again in vogue. The posticheurs who advertise in the great French journals remodelled all their designs, which previously had been waved and curled, and the *calots* and turbans were in every case represented as nearly straight.

Naturally, the ladies' hairdressers are greatly annoyed; but, helped this time by their leading clients, they are combatting this horrible fashion, which all the workgirls and rank and file amongst the public of Paris have promptly adopted.

The Fashion for 1910

The '*calot*' effectively supplanted the curled chignons, which, by their dainty lightness, were very appropriate for waved headdresses. The turban, too, by its ample proportions, nearly choked all demand for waving.

But let the Trade not become despondent at the prospect; the present coiffure is becoming general too rapidly for it to have any chance of permanence.

A careful survey of the new creations in millinery of our leading establishments, and also of the coiffures executed at the great Paris hairdressing function of 19th December last, enables me to say that the fashion in hair for next spring will somewhat resemble the mode adopted during the French Revolution by the celebrated woman-painter of the time, Mme. Lebrun.

To sum up, I may state that the turban shows clear evidences of decline in Paris because there was never anything artistic about it, and because it has become common and odious and was always prejudicial to the real commercial interests of the Hairdressing Trade.

Waving, always gracious and beautiful, will modernise the new coiffure a little and should retain for the hairdresser the feminine *clientèle* who were on the verge of leaving him.

February 5, 1910: The Influence of Millinery on Hairdressing Fashions in Paris

Hairdressers, as I believe I have already said, do not create fashions, they submit to them. The present coiffure, for instance, would probably never have existed had it not been for the gigantic, bell-shaped hats – the sort of extinguishers which envelope not only the hair by almost the whole of the head.

The leading Parisian modistes [milliners] – those who appropriate to their select circle the valuable patronage of the elegant aristocracy – are all situated in the Rue de la Paix or the Rue Royal. In place of shops they occupy splendid suites of apartments, the annual rental of which varies between 25,000 and 100,000 francs (£1,000–4,000). I could mention one suite in which the reception salon alone cost for decoration and equipment 125,000 francs. It is scarcely necessary to add that these modistes have what in England would be termed 'sleeping partners,' most of whom are purveyors of expensive feathers, flowers and other accessories.

All these '*marchandes de modes*,' as they were called in the Louis XVI period pay their attentions to the women and ruin the husbands, so ingenious are they in creating business by continually varying their creations, and making their seductiveness over-powering. One finds at their establishments hats for which as much as 1,500 each is asked; the models at 1,000 francs are quite ordinary, and should a client's request be for 'a morning hat' at 150 francs, the saleswoman will not even trouble to serve her. These modistes never concern themselves about the coiffeur – he might not even exist; and yet it is within their power to enrich or to ruin him.

I may, however, remark in passing, that there are in Paris some hairdressers whose turnovers per annum are commencing to attract attention, since one of them – M. Georges, Rue Royale – has just sold his business to a company for the fancy sum of 600,000 francs. But let us continue.

By the time that this article is published straw hats will have made their appearance in Paris, for our capital is always well in advance of the time. Already the modistes are occupied in devising and perfecting their creations for next winter, and here is an idea of what is occurring in the establishment of Mme. Caroline Reboux:

The female designers, who during the year frequently visit the museums and libraries in order to collect the necessary documents, have just submitted their ideas and designs. Their aim, of course, is to suggest radical alterations in style, because largest sales are absolutely necessary, and in order to sell much it is imperative that the models should be continually altered. Mme. Reboux, therefore, called together recently all the leading designers. She explained the nature and form of hat that she desired introduced, supplied them with documents to aid them, and allotted to each a period of eight days within which to produce five or six models of this kind. But the greatest latitude is allowed to the designers in all that concerns the embellishment and details of ornamentation; they have even *carte blanche* to purchase, make, or develop, no matter at what cost, any ornaments and accessories which appear to them necessary.

Here are the completed models, each bearing a label on which is written the cost price and a number corresponding to the name of the creator. Mme. Reboux accepts them all, as if she had no opinion herself, and exhibits them in a special apartment, while those who have produced them take a fortnight's holiday, well rewarded.

Then, on the invitation of the great modiste, the fashion introducers come to see and to try the new styles, and they choose the ones which please them most; they freely contribute their opinions, and ask sometimes for modifications – a request to which the greatest heed is paid.

It will already be understood that I mean by 'fashion introducers' the ladies Letellier, Marthe Régnier, Ludvine, Arlette Dorgère, Robine, etc. – that is to say, all the pretty and elegant women, all the theatrical celebrities of Paris, to whom the modistes and dressmakers do not generally represent their accounts, because the fees on the other hand for exhibiting their creations are very considerable.

In France, under the monarchy or under the Empire, fashion emanated from the Court. Under the Republic, it is the queens of beauty or of celebrity who select the hats that they desire to wear, and it is they who really set the fashions – on the summer racecourse; at the smart resorts of the winter, such as the skating rinks, the theatres, the select five o'clock tea parties; the *salons de peinture* of the spring; the horse shows of the autumn; or, finally, the fashionable restaurants at all seasons of the year. It is then that the representatives of the great French and foreign houses can see the fashions of Paris; and it is then that the modistes of the second class and the large drapery establishments[3] commence to copy the models and to disseminate them amongst the general public.

But by this time the grand modiste of the Rue de la Paix has already reaped a rich harvest, and the fortunate creators of the selected modes have also derived ample recompense for their efforts.

So long as the milliners continue to wield their present influence over fashionable women and succeed in retaining their allegiance for the great variety of their creations, so long will the hairdresser occupy a secondary position. The *salon* of the great modiste of to-day is, to elegant ladies, what the mirror of the sportsman is to the lark. They are all attracted there as by an irresistible compelling force, and they listen as to an oracle and believe without questioning. One has only to go there with a client, as I have done myself, to understand it.

'That hat suits you, does it not, madame?' says the great modiste. 'Ah! in order that it may be adapted still more to your features, it is necessary to pull it down over the eyes, to straighten your hair in front and to dress your hair bulgingly at back.'

The thing is done! The modiste has spoken, and the hairdresser has nothing more to say. There only remains to us the duty of making what is required, and to bow our heads before the superior power.

March 5, 1910: A Device for 'Lengthening' Hair

Since the middle of the year 1909, when the fashion of long hair came into vogue, it has been generally found that fine and lengthy hair has been rare and costly; on the other hand, the Institut des Coiffeurs de Dames de France,[4] which has an Arbitration and Expert Committee connected with the Justices of the Peace, has been much agitated by the fact that not a single day has passed without this Committee finding it necessary to intervene in order to regulate judicial matters arising out of complaints made by clients against their hairdressers on the subject of Chinese hair, which the latter had sold to them. For my part, I have on an average five complaints of this kind to

---

3. That is, department stores.
4. A group of the most eminent ladies' hairdressers in Paris, of which Long was the general secretary.

examine every week, and to my great regret I am nearly always obliged to decide against my colleagues who sell as first quality hair horrible Oriental stuff, badly dyed and clumsily prepared.

Ultimately, in the face of these repeated complaints, the members of our Institut were compelled to seek a remedy. But the idea which was unanimously adjudged the best was that of our esteemed colleague, M. Perrin, which I propose to describe.

Monsieur Perrin is as respected as he is well-known amongst the Trade workers of Paris; he has invented numerous Trade devices from which we have all derived benefit. In his hard struggle for existence, M. Perrin's beard turned prematurely white, but he harbours no rancour against destiny, for his motto is that of our mutualist – 'One for all and all for one.' He is, indeed, the least selfish of men, since he has allowed his most recent Trade invention to be exploited in the name of the Institut, of which he is the doyen, M. Perrin has registered in the name of 'Marie-Louis' his barrette and pins, which have been specially protected in order to preserve their ownership.

The 'Marie-Louise' device consists simply of a barrette pierced with little holes into which is sewn a length of clubbed hair or two lengths [permitting short locks of hair to be connected seamlessly. It allows for the use of hair] obtainable cheaply, ornamented pleasingly and as long as may be desired to encircle the head for a coiffure *à la mode*. It can be seen how ingenious this invention is and what service it can render to us in the struggle against the competition of the big drapery houses. I advise my colleagues not to hesitate in using it until the device is taken up by the bazaars.

April 2, 1910: A Revival of the 'Coque Normande'

Those young French hairdressers who suddenly became ladies' hands because of waving and who have succeeded in earning a fairly comfortable living for several years simply by waving the hair, are now finding themselves almost without work.

At first they were much surprised at this sudden change, being unable to attribute it to anything, but they are beginning to understand now that the fashion which necessitates 'dressing' is returning and they are in despair, being completely ignorant of this 'new style.'

The reason is that you can no more become a 'hairdresser' suddenly, than you can at once become a 'waver.' 'Hairdressing,' properly called, requires special study and long practice, the same as 'waving,' and although each may be considered on a level with each other, the two specialities are quite distinct.

The young people I referred to had not considered that, nor had they given a thought to the morrow; they neither took the trouble to get ready for a possible change nor to reflect on the perpetual evolution that goes on in regard to style as well as professional methods. That is why everything appears to them to be 'new.'

But really there is nothing new in the proper acceptation of the word; we renovate frequently, we transform and refresh, but we get nothing, or very little, that is actually new. It is easy to give proof of this in regard to hairdressing and postiche. Everything which is being done as 'new' at the present time has already been done by past generations.

And yet these renowned forerunners had not the help of our modern improvements. But they had the advantage of really good practical training, having served complete apprenticeships with resolute masters. Their day's work was nearly double the length of ours, for they were not afraid of working in the gas-light, and even till one hour after midnight, when necessary, always in the company of their masters, who fulfilled at the same time the rôle of teacher and educator. Thus the sentiment of the art gradually developed itself in them, the sentiment without which the ladies' hand cannot succeed.

These and many other things in honour of the hairdressers of former times were admirably expressed in Paris on March 10th, by Monsieur Perrin, in the course of a debate, organised by the *Capilartiste*,[5] between himself (representing the École Classique), and a young colleague who personified the École Moderne. Then, in the course of another discourse by Monsieur Stéphane,[6] illustrated by 100 lantern slides, the hairdressing and celebrated hairdressers of different periods were awarded suitable tributes.

For my own part, I will limit myself now to recalling that in 1865 people wore, as in the present day, turbans – that is to say, voluminous chignons mounted on a vast whalebone mount, and dressed uniformly straight, with interlacings of the hair in coques, or in curls, under the general name of 'Coque Normande,' and we now witness its return with pleasure, under other names, but almost the same thing. It will be observed that they are all surmounted by magnificent combs, such as are not made nowadays, because customers who would spend £8 [200 francs] for a similar article, in shell with designs and incrustations of fine gold (or set in fine gold) are now rather few.

5. The trade paper, of which Long was founder and editor.
6. The famous Belgian coiffeur, who served Queen Elizabeth of Belgium, among other celebrities.

May 7, 1910: The Low Coiffure is Returning Slowly but Surely

It is now nearly thirty years since the hairdressers of Paris were longing for the return of the low coiffure, and since then they have individually made many praiseworthy but vain efforts to accomplish their desire.

At different times we have seen here and there a few persons wearing their chignons on the neck, because that was their individual style of dressing their hair; but it can be rightly said that the fashion that we all wish to see in vogue, because of its being commercially more favourable to our Trade, has not been made at all general. Why?

The low head-dress had no chance of being adopted for day wear because the collars to the dresses were too high. Such details as these are well known to those of us, who, in order to be well-informed, and in a position to analyse the latest tendencies of fashion, have to be continually interviewing and conferring with the leading supply houses of Paris. We have even made several applications to the principal dressmakers with the view of getting them to reduce the height of the bodices. At last this has now been done. With the advent of spring, the high collars have disappeared, to make way for smart low collarettes. The curls, therefore, can descend little by little on to the neck, then extend so far as the nape, and later on – although this may be rather a long way off yet – convey their soft caresses to the uncovered shoulders, at the playhouse or at the ball.

Moreover, it is now clear that the curled and waved turban has triumphed over the *calot* with straight, smooth hair. The ladies' hairdressers of Paris are again deriving some revenue from the short curls, either by making fringes, or in the form of voluminous chignons.

We can only hope that this new mode will become definitely established, for the curls entail waving and the low coiffure stimulates the sale of a good deal of postiche. Moreover, the large drapery emporiums cannot make curled postiche, as they can plaits and other straight hairwork. There is some prospect, therefore, of better days in store for the Trade, and certainly a little relief from the stress of outside competition and recent dull business conditions will be very welcome.

June 4, 1910: After the Turban

A very fortunate thing for ladies' hairdressers has been the abandonment by ladies of fashion of the ball-shaped coiffure, dressed with straight hair, which was more often than not sold by the drapery establishments. In any case, with this kind of coiffure ladies no longer had any need of the hairdresser, and so did not visit our shops, or very seldom; they did not require to ask us to attend on them at their residences; and consequently we were unable to sell them anything. The sale of shell combs, perfumes, and hair ornaments, and even of false hair, went to the stores.

Here is a reason, therefore, why the attention of the whole Trade should be directed to the importance of inventing something special, which will force customers to come to us, and which will compel them to come again, or to claim our services constantly. Even if this were not lucrative in itself, it would become advantageous indirectly, for when we attend on a lady, we gain by the opportunity this provides for effecting sales.

Marcel, in creating his waving, discovered this 'special thing,' which assured us direct contact with our feminine clientèle and which ushered in an epoch of great prosperity for the hairdresser. So long as the Marcel wave was at its height, we heard nothing of our redoubtable competitors; but as soon as the turban appeared (with *straight* hair) the stores quickly snatched up our business, it being easy for them to hold huge stocks of this class of goods.

Now that light, soft hairdressing is returning, the stores are perturbed. They are no longer able to pile up the right sort of hair; it is much more delicate and requires far more room, necessitating also constant care and even the frequent intervention of the hair-preparer.

With the reign of straight hair, the profane merchants triumph, with the advent of curled and waved hair ladies return to the hairdresser.

It is in our interest, therefore, to aim at maintaining soft, fluffy tresses; all our efforts must, for the moment, be brought to bear on this essential point, and as we are much more numerous than the drapery houses, it cannot be doubted that, if hairdressers will persistently apply their activities and influence in this direction, the result will be satisfactory to our Trade.

July 2, 1910: Curled Postiche and Waved Postiche

Taking the point of view of an ordinary ladies' hand, and starting with the idea that postiche is the profitable basis of hairdressing, I will endeavour to dress a coiffure elegantly with simple postiche.

Under the conditions which now prevail – the assortment of raw materials offered by our supply houses, the aid of our journals and special books, the demonstrations in the evening schools, etc. – there should not be a single coiffeur who does not make up postiche. The man who commences this branch and only deals in rudimentary articles, is still very useful to customers of limited means, who are always more numerous than the others; he also

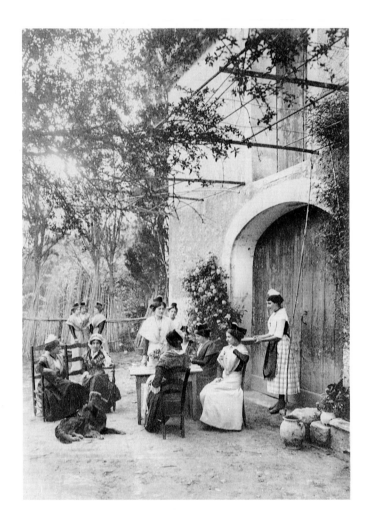

Figure 2. 'Hair Harvest in the village of Saint-Rémy-en-Provence.' From Jeanne de
Flandreysey, *La femme provençale* (Marseille: F. Détaille, 1922).

imparts a taste for postiche to persons who could not afford to go to a tiptop posticheur, and who henceforward will spend a little more in order to have something 'a little better' every time. Moreover, these people will be kept from the drapery establishment, and there's the rub! The more posticheurs there are the more clients there will be for postiche. Hairdressing gives to the hairdresser his daily bread. Postiche rids us of the slavery attaching to continual shaving; it makes us like our trade because it procures us ease; it permits us to know more about the hair of which so many of our colleagues are ignorant. It exercises our taste and imagination by the variety of its styles and the need of creating others; it teaches us slowly but surely how to handle hair and to make rational coiffures by the study of the successive stages. In effect, it may be said that each piece of postiche represents a part of a coiffure, and that, as with everything else, the detail must be known before the whole can be constructed.

August 6, 1910: The Coiffure of Light Curl

Now that the dead season is reigning in Paris, hairdressers do not incur much expense in setting out their windows; consequently it cannot be said with certainty what will be the precise innovations of the next season. There may be some surprises, but it seems that the tendency is towards the curled headdress.

In the sixteenth century a number of fashionable ladies allowed their hair to be cut in order that they might be able to wear the curled coiffure, which was then greatly in favour. Two centuries later, Queen Marie Antoinette, losing her hair after her *accouchement* [having given birth], had it cut fairly short, and she wore the curled head-dress (children's style), which the grand ladies of the epoch also adopted. Under the Consulate which followed the great French Revolution [1799–1804], ladies again resorted to the process of cutting their hair, and this time with the intention of wearing it straight, but in face of the ugly simplicity of the coiffures, they soon had their hair curled as well. Not so long ago, the last generation of ladies' hairdressers were acquainted with the celebrated coiffure 'à la Ninon,' for which the hair was cut and curled. Finally, the curled head-dress has prevailed in our own time, in certain places where the women do not disdain to give themselves the airs of a boy. For this reason, this coiffure is to-day looked upon as unladylike.

Naturally, if the curled head-dress does become the fashion again it will not have an unladylike appearance; it will be re-established in the public mind and adopted by the majority. In any case, no matter what fate is reserved for it, let it be said at once that the coiffure of light curls bears but a very distant resemblance to the old-time style.

Firstly, the modern hairdresser no longer requests a client to sacrifice the most beautiful of Nature's adornments; to-day we should consider it a crime of lèse-beauty to pass the scissors over a healthy head of hair. Again, to daily curl the short hair was possible in the olden times, when things went more slowly, but not to-day when everybody is in a hurry and everything is done so rapidly, thanks to modern mechanical improvements and electricity. For the rest, cut hair can neither remain permanently curled, nor give a very elegant coiffure in spite of the skill of the dresser.

Modern postiche having attained a high degree of perfection, we are able to counteract the drawbacks mentioned in the previous paragraph; it is with postiche that we are going to execute this new coiffure. It remains to be seen what form this postiche will take – whether wigs or other large pieces; elaborate and complicated or otherwise. But do not let us overlook the fact that nothing is better than simplicity; there is in that much which we have too long ignored.

I have often remarked in the course of my travels that the difference between Parisian artisans and others is that the former know admirably how to 'present' their work. Whether the work done be that of furniture, dresses, or anything else, the articles will, perhaps, be made less summarily, but the finish of the furniture and the chic appearance of the dresses will be incomparable. No doubt the same thing applies in regard to postiche, and if my foreign colleagues think that this is the case, they must see to it that they take very great pains in the dressing of the postiche.

September 3, 1910: Hairdressing Fantastic and Comic

This is, indeed, an age of surprises. I certainly was prepared for practically anything from the caprices of Fashion, but what has happened is beyond even my wildest anticipations.

Having spent a few days in quietude at the *chateau* of my illustrious friend, Marcel, on the route to Trouville, the most frequented of French watering places, I adopted the practice of going there during the afternoon, in order to take note of the latest coiffures of the elegant and eccentric Parisiennes. What I observed there was scarcely credible – young women, handsome, wealthy or lavishly provided for, whom everybody looks at and aspires to imitate, and who so far succeeded in making themselves conspicuous that they incited public laughter. Some of them wore costumes cut very short and so narrow round the legs as to make it scarcely possible for one foot to be

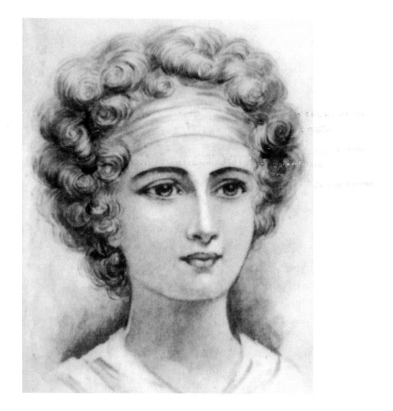

Figure 3. The 'Clown' Coiffure. From *HWJS*, September 3, 1910.

put before the other; others had hats as voluminous as umbrellas, or, at the other extreme, small woollen caps which fitted very closely to the head. But what interested me most of all was to see these ladies at the moment when they were bareheaded. Believe me, I do not exaggerate when I say that, having discarded the parting, these women now dress their hair after the style of clowns.

Returning to Paris, still full of wonderment at what I had seen at Trouville-on-Sea, I have found that there are already here not a few 'clownesses' – at the theatres, the swell restaurants, in the Champs-Elysées, Bois de Boulogne, etc. The French and English newspapers have begun to write about this new and comical coiffure. One of our *confrères* in the Boulevard Haussmann has even thus early exhibited in his window a figure with the hair dressed in this style.

All this proves that this *fantasie* of bad taste is not confined to the eccentric people one encounters at Trouville, but constitutes a clear tendency of fashion, of which we as up-to-date coiffeurs must take due note.

If this style should become general, it will not be merely a few pieces of postiche that will be necessary to dress the coiffure, but complete wigs – yes, curled wigs as worn by the aristocratic folk in past centuries – whilst others less elegant must have their hair cut, and frizzed and curled daily with the hot iron.

In olden times the duration of a coiffure covered a very long period, but little by little the time was reduced. Under Napoleon I, Fashion had already begun to wane after about a year; then, at the period when Marcel introduced his waving, the styles changed every three months. To-day one is considered out of fashion if a particular coiffure is worn for a month.

To mechanical production and the stress of competition must be attributed this rapidity of change. Under these conditions it would not be, perhaps, inadvisable for the hairdresser-posticheur to endeavour to modernise his plant, to improve his system of production, and to amend his commercial methods according to present-day requirements. Far be it from me to express words of criticism regarding any of my colleagues, but truly there exist far too many who are hindrances to progress. And this is why the large drapery houses, and others, stand so little on ceremony, but one after the other appropriate to their establishments articles which are incontestably within our province.

Let us put aside our prejudices and jealousies; let us jointly work for the maintenance and improvement of the sources of income which are ours by right; and then I have no doubt that in the end we shall be the winners in the severe economic conflict which now threatens to overwhelm the small shop-keeper.

October 1, 1910: What Will be Worn This Winter

The above is the traditional question with which ladies' hairdressers and posticheurs are confronted at the commencement of each season. My readers have, no doubt, already put the question, or heard it put, for our elegant clients ask it often enough when we are least expecting it. In this event, woe betide the man who stutters out a few vague generalities, or who is imprudent enough to reply: 'I don't know; I think a little of everything will be worn!' That hairdresser immediately loses at least three things – (1) the customer's confidence; (2) the profit on one or several transactions; and (3) his part in the artistic prestige of his Trade. To this unfortunate coiffeur the lady might reply: 'But the bootmaker cannot tell me the style in hairdressing. In any case I shall consult another hairdresser in the future one who is better acquainted with the events of his profession.'

Therefore, always have an answer ready; do not allow yourself to be taken by surprise. If you cannot give good reasons, you should rather give bad ones than give none at all. It is a thousand times better to pass for a man who has deceived himself, rather than for one who does not know. Especially in matters of fashion and the toilet, where tastes and preferences are so divided, should you be affirmative; you should know how to sustain a subject, no matter what, in order to attract notice. But what is still more preferable, of course, is to have an opinion with some foundation, one that is backed up with proofs from some good source.

November 4, 1910: The Coming of the Toque and its Influence on Fashions in Hair

The struggle which continually exists between the ladies' hairdresser and his client has just assumed an acute character, and, foreseeing our own defeat, I return to the question.

'He who pays the piper calls the tune!' The lady who pays to have her hair dressed has a right to see her tastes and desires triumphant. Twenty years ago, when Marcel waving was at its height, those who refused to wave their clients' hair saw themselves pitilessly abandoned by the public; two years ago, when the great demand for Marcel waving suddenly ceased, those who refused to do anything but waving also lost their connection.

After these experiences I advise my colleagues not to be obstinate and hug to themselves the notion that fashion will not change. Fashion in coiffures does change continuously, and at present the change tends in its general form towards smaller proportions. Already the actresses and *demi-mondaines* of Paris, who always exert great influence over Fashion, are wearing little or no postiche; the better middle-class folk use a fair amount of postiche, while the fashionable section of the working class wear a good deal of it.

Before applying any remedy [the Institut] sought out the source of the trouble. I had the honour, in company with our eminent colleague, M. Perrin, to make enquiries amongst the greatest of the Parisian modistes. 'What are you preparing for the season?' we asked the chiefs of these important firms, and the reply everywhere was, 'toques – toques in velvet, and in furs of all kinds.' 'Why are you giving a preference to toques?' 'We do not make toques out of preference, but simply because our hat-shapers have been on strike for four months and we cannot procure felt shapes.'

Therefore, toques are to be worn, and with them coiffures not too voluminous in extent, so that they may be capable of accommodating the toques.

Whilst we were with the great modistes I [observed] those who try on the hats, or toques for the lady clients to see. It goes without saying that these young ladies are very elegant, that they dress their hair to suit the needs of their business, and that they are very frequently imitated, and in adopting the hat, the clients also copy the arrangement of the hair. All of these saleswomen have their hair waved more or less all round the head. These women invariably have a small form of headdress, but, notwithstanding, they nearly all wear postiche.

December 3, 1910: The Difference Between the Coiffure which is Passing and that Which is Coming

Last month I explained to readers what ought to be the *coiffure du jour* to suit the fashionable hats, and especially the toques – for the coiffures worn by ladies nowadays do not keep within the bounds of merely sustaining the hats, they penetrate them. I have said that fashionable ladies of Paris prefer the small coiffures worn by the artistes and saleswomen at the big millinery establishments to the voluminous headdresses persisted in by the coiffeur. In this matter, the victory certainly lies at the door of the client, for it is she who pays, and pays to see her taste triumphant. On the other hand, the hairdresser is not at all indispensable to her.

Last year the general shape was large and bulky. The volume was especially pronounced at the top and rear of the coiffure. At this the end of the year, the volume has disappeared. The head-dresses are small, or relatively so. Persons of taste are in agreement that with robes so narrow ladies cannot have their hair dressed in a wide formation without violating the most elementary rules of aestheticism. Moreover, as we have said, the present style of hat does not permit of a voluminous arrangement of the hair. The vast chignons of curls are no longer seen except upon the heads of less fashionable ladies, who get their ideas and supplies from the drapery establishments.

In short, very wide waves, very wide strands of hair, and very wide pins for rather small coiffures – these are the conspicuous features of modern hairdressing.

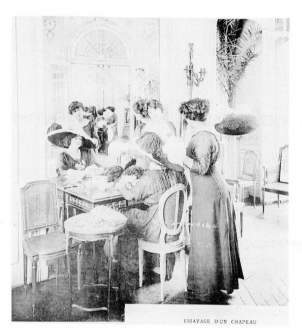

ESSAYAGE D'UN CHAPEAU

Figure 4. 'Essayage d'un chapeau.' Elite clients trying on the latest hats. From Editions du Figaro, *Les créateurs de la mode* (Paris: Ch. Eggemann, 1910).

2

1911

January 7, 1911: The Coiffure with Two Partings

Now a word about ornaments for the hair, which, like everything else, are continually changing. One of the happiest ideas of the season has come from our colleague, Monsieur Perrin, who has to his credit so many Trade inventions. His system is to attach to the rigid bandeaux of the nape, much in vogue at this moment, two strands of hair to encircle the coiffure. These two strands are mounted squarely and attached to the shaped or decorated bandeaux by means of M. Perrin's 'Marie-Louise' barrette. It would be difficult to over-estimate the services which can be rendered by this accessory: half postiche, half ornament. Firstly, it avoids thicknesses, which are always inconvenient and disagreeable in a relatively small headdress, as is preferred at the present time by our fashionable clients. It also constitutes a novelty, and that is usually sufficient for ladies to adopt it, for novelties are very rare – as rare as they are lucrative.

Another innovation that may be mentioned is the revival of aigrettes and high feathers in the ornamentation of theatre coiffures. I would not like my readers to think that this style is general, nor even possible for all ladies, because of the decided movement against large hats and ornaments, but [such ornaments are] now worn on Fridays by many very fashionable ladies in their own boxes at the Opera, where, of course, they annoy nobody.

Finally, I may add that one has never before seen in Paris such pretty or such rich hair ornaments as are now conspicuous. That is accounted for by the fact that the artist-designers, collaborating with the leading ladies hairdressers and certain *brodeurs d'art* [embroiderers], have produced some elaborate designs, which are sold at prices as high as 300 francs each. The best Parisian women workers are making the designs of the artists on skins and leathers of all shades, on the richest stuffs, with golden threads and multicoloured silks and with precious stones, costly pearls, and fine spangles. The *brodeuses* in question are devoting as much as a month's work to a single ornament. The jewellers and shellworkers are likewise devising remarkable productions for the ornamentation of the feminine head.

February 4, 1911: Paris Novelties: The 'Mysterious' Chignons

There are times when the coiffure is extremely simple; at others it is very complicated, and the one form usually follows the other. Without attempting to cite far-fetched examples, I may recall that before the advent of Marcel waving (which simplified hairdressing to a great extent) women wore masses of switches and plaits of Chinese hair, which were not only very heavy, but were also disposed of in inextricable confusion. Still more recently, only three or four years ago, it required more than an hour to wave, separate the puffy portions, frizz and arrange them. Then there were garlands and bunches of curls, which had to be previously dressed with the fingers; afterwards a ribbon was interlaced in the coiffure, a net was placed, the whole shape of the head-dress was adjusted, combs were inserted, together with a barrette for the neck, and, finally, some fancy pins. Parisiennes used certainly to get something for their money when they required all that for an average of 2 francs. For, I should add, that it was only in shops where they used to dress cheaply that the coiffure was complicated. And this exaggeration brought about its own downfall, in which, of course, we have the experience of life – when a man has mounted high enough, and arrived at the summit, he must come down! The turban, which was afterwards in vogue, brought us near to the simplicity of primitive times.

But this great simplicity could not last either; its attractive power waned rapidly, and it was replaced by enormous chignons of curls, which have already been discarded. Fashionable clients abandon all postiche that can be bought cheaply at any drapery store, and return to the specialist – to him who knows his trade, who alone can give a personal touch to the coiffure of his client, as distinct from that of the chambermaid and the shop girl. A lady cannot, of course, dress her hair in the same style as do her servants, seeing that she can afford more both in her postiche and toilet as well as for her hats. And besides the question of expense, there is that of style, which must of necessity be kept distinct. A fashionable lady may adopt a mode which is not worn by everybody, but she changes this as soon as she sees herself copied by someone who appears to be inferior to her socially.

March 4, 1911: What is the Tendency of Fashion?

The theatre? Let us not pay any heed to the fantasies of bad taste that are to be seen there. In order that their headdresses may be different from others, women may be seen at the theatre wearing coiffures of the most absurd and eccentric description. Yak wigs are resorted to in imitation of powdered coiffures, and often one sees Persian bonnets, Dutch headgear, Venetian linen caps, plumes, flowers, aigrettes, gaudy jewellry, red caps as worn during the French Revolution, with golden tassels – all used in profusion, without taste or discretion, and constituting a veritable masquerade.

Can it be that from these carnival effects Fashion is to emerge? Surely not.

I am hoping, and with confidence, that there will occur something like a revolution in costumes, in manners and customs, in politics – in fact, in anything that will rid us of this state of anarchy, for undoubtedly hairdressing is in the mire and can only free itself by a complete revolution. The sooner that occurs the better; we have little to lose and everything to gain by a radical change, whatever the form it may assume.

In present circumstances, the hairdresser derives little benefit; ladies have practically no more need for our services, for they are dressing their own coiffures with the straight hair which they purchased last year and very probably at a drapery house. In order to effect the sale of an expensive transformation, or of postiche of any value, it is not now sufficient that one should supply a good article, or be a clever salesman; it is almost necessary to execute what I may call a commercial acrobatic feat.

Amongst the leaders of fashion, the generalization of the harem skirt is a matter of moment. It is not, perhaps, a nice introduction, but it has something of a practical nature in these days of sport and aviation. After the harem skirt will come the masculine waistcoat, with platron, and thereafter we many easily arrive at the boy coiffure, so much wished for by some ladies.

Whilst gentlemen are permitting their hair to grow in order that they may curl and dress it after the style of 1830, ladies will cut theirs, so that they may curl it, too, and so contribute to the equalisation of the sexes, which is their dream and ambition. When that day arrives wigs will be worn and our Trade will be saved. From the small wig we shall soon pass to the big one – and why not?

April 1911: The Form of the Coiffure is always Subordinate to the Fashion in Hats

When one is desirous of securing reliable guidance as to the form of the modern coiffure, knowledge and inspiration can readily be abstracted from the shape of the fashionable millinery, for the one cannot exist without the other. I therefore conclude that some information as to the tendency of the latest creations in hats will be of interest and help.

Well, the new hats offered to the parisiennes this springtime are of two

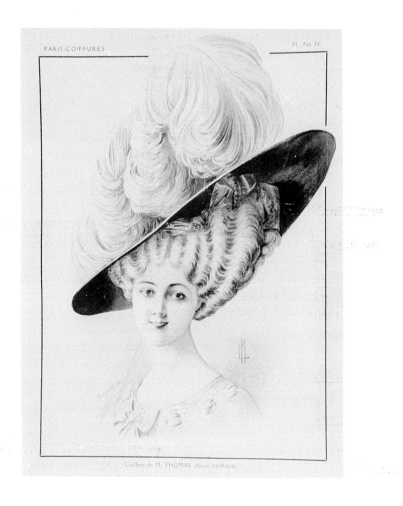

PARIS-COIFFURES

Pl. No IV.

Coiffure de M. THOMAS (Maison GRIMAUD)

Figure 5. Coiffure by M. Thomas. From *Paris-Coiffures*, 1908–9.

kinds – very large or very small; there is no medium. The very large ones are almost flat, so that they allow ladies to show a little of their hair. As to the others, they will continue to extend right down to the shoulders, with a few exceptions. It was at the first races at Auteuil[1] – where the most fashionable people of the season meet. The Napoleon style predominates, and although

1. The fashionable race course at the western edge of Paris.

this shape in itself does not lack prettiness, it can be imagined that it will not be to our advantage. The coiffures that are possible with these hats will be pointed, like sugar loaves and somewhat voluminous. There is, again, a clearly-marked tendency to entirely cover the ears; in fact, ladies seem to be annoyed if they cannot show their hair – they free it as much as they are able from these strange hats, which savour more of fancy dress than of novelty.

For observant coiffeurs it is always useful to frequent fashionable gatherings, and all those who wish to keep to the front should adopt this practice, like the modistes and dressmakers, in order to note the tendency of fashion. Personally, I observed that the colours of the hats and dresses were always bright, and, for preference, cherry-red or green. This will be a useful indication in regard to the choice of ornaments, ribbons, etc.

Another and no less important point is that blond hair, and especially artificial blond, obtained by oxygenated water (hydrogen peroxide) is no longer fashionable. The mahogany red is becoming more and more dark and the browns triumph. It is very fortunate for us that the black hennas in powder and paste have been discovered.

[At Auteuil] I also noticed some coiffures without postiche, waved by means of curl papers and made excessively glossy, according to the style of about 1830–1840. Of course, the hair was brown and the wearers were paid to exhibit certain creations of the dressmakers. It is well known that these latter insist on their mannequins [models] wearing small coiffures.

July 1911: Bonnets of Lace and Bonnets of Hair. The Latest Postiche in Paris

Each of us knows quite well how difficult it becoming to maintain business on account of over production and of the great competition existing in every branch of our industry; it follows, therefore, that each, in his own line, makes strenuous attempts to secure the adoption of his products or models. In Paris especially, where general expenses are enormous, one does not know what to create or what to invent in order to appeal to the fashionable *clientèle*. The time has long gone by when the hairdresser troubled himself about whether that which he was introducing was in good taste or answered to a need; now he is constantly devising, modifying and transforming with the one object of drawing away from his neighbour clients who have money to spend.

The coiffeur is lamenting because he has been ruined by the modiste; by creating a demand for bee-hive hats, which reach down to the shoulders, the

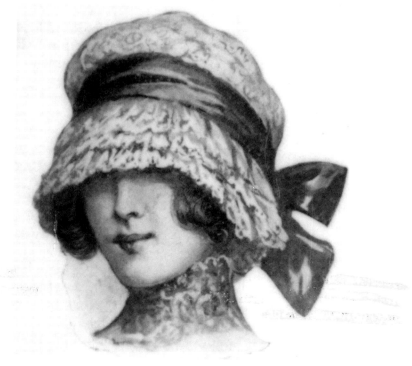

Figure 6. Lace Bonnet. From *HWJS*, July 1911.

milliner has killed waving, hairdressing and postiche, because they are useless to the majority of women. And, in turn, the modiste is now going to find himself dethroned by the dealer in lingerie. It is rumoured in well-informed circles that bonnets are to replace the ordinary hats. A quantity of them have already been seen on racecourses which are frequented by the *élite* of the fashionable world, which signifies that they have been launched in high society circles.

Certainly the bonnet is not a novelty, but probably such rich or valuable ones have never been seen before; the finest embroidery and rarest lace adorn these new models, the least costly of which run to several hundred francs. It is obvious that at that price the wives of the people will not be able to indulge, but the big drapery establishments are watching this article, and having prepared themselves to imitate it at a low price, they will soon be sending out some thousands of samples.

We revolted, so to speak against the hats which almost hid the hair; what shall we do now if this new mode takes on, seeing that it allows of no hair being shown at all?

Most fortunately for us there is a fairly large section of our lady customers who do not like such extravagance in their headgear, and who only adopt such eccentric styles in the last extremity; they will doubtless remain faithful to us for a long time yet. There are some even who could not do without the services of a coiffeur, nor the help of a well-made postiche.

When I speak of different dimensions in postiche, I do so not without reason. For some time past – from the moment that the big drapery establishments captured the sale of false hair, or rather of the small classical pieces which are easy to make up and to stock, such as tails, torsades, plaits and curls – since then the master posticheurs of Paris have busied themselves with devising more advantageous models – more important, more difficult to keep in perfect condition. They have apparently succeeded in following the example first set by M. Marius Heng with his 'Sans-Gène,' his 'Sans-Souci,' and his 'Sans-Pareil.' These are complete coiffures mounted on a kind of frame, which is placed on the head all complete, exactly like an ordinary bonnet.

It will be seen, therefore, that the exploitation of the 'bonnet' of hair, which I have just described, and which, of course, may be dressed in all sorts of ways, will compensate to a great extent for the disastrous effects of the lace bonnet to which I referred at the beginning of this article.

August 1911: New Postiche for Covering the Ears

I have already referred in previous articles to the shapes of ladies' hats, which govern, so to speak, the headdress and the postiche worn. I have also indicated that this season, apart from the very large hats, which are the most fashionable, the majority of ladies only wear small models, similar to the hat of a pierrot, or to that of a colonial. These fit so far over the head that parisiennes no longer have any need for hat pins, which have become superfluous since the headgear goes on the head like a coif or wig. It is this detail which has banished curls from the *coiffure de ville*.

But the ladies have not been slow to discover that they look less pretty like this than with a little hair showing around the face. It is useless to invent things which are too far removed from the laws of nature. By implanting hair on the forehead, Nature not only intended to protect the head, but also to provide a charming framework for our physiognomies. The most uncivilised barbarians and savages preserve their hair intact and attach the greatest importance to it.

It is therefore plainly our duty to inform clients that they will never look so becoming as when showing their hair. This is what Parisian coiffeurs are doing at the present time; and the ladies, signifying their agreement, are adopting a kind of knot, or small bunch of curls, which extends on to the temples and even a little on to the cheeks, and is quite visible under their hats or bonnets of lace.

September 1911: Characteristic Tendencies of Ladies Hairdressing

As I informed my colleagues the 'Ninoche' hats have resulted in (1) the adoption of flat-topped coiffures, (2) the generalisation of the centre parting, and (3) the advancing of the bandeaux on to the cheeks. When it is not the flat bandeaux which are brought forward, it is the curls or knots, which are being worn in front of the ears.

In order to obtain a good idea as to whether this style of coiffure was exceptional, I have for a month kept careful observation on the world of fashion in several centres. Unfortunately, the example having been set by the fashionable world, it has spread like wild-fire. It was *la belle Sorel*[2] – usually three centuries old in her adopted fashions – who took to raising her hair thus during last July, and her example has been much copied since. As a rule, when a fashion that is so prejudicial to our Trade's interests threatens to spread we endeavour to discover a Mlle. Lantelme, that pretty and attractive girl, the spoilt child of the Parisians, who has just perished, unfortunately, by drowning in the Rhine. This actress was not only extremely handsome; she pleased the public very much, and the public often copied what she wore. In this way the ladies' hairdressers brought some influence to bear on the modes. At present, however, I cannot see anybody who will replace Lantelme for her beauty, and especially for her willingness to hold herself at our disposal with such good grace and beneficial effect.

October 1911: In Favour of the 'Low' Chignon

In spite of all our efforts, the fashion in hair of the last two years has been unfavourable to us – that is to say, since ladies of fashion declared war on the abuse of waving and curls as seen on the heads of their servants, and adopted the straight coiffure and the horrible turban. From that time the big drapery establishments have competed very seriously with us by retailing straight hair, the only kind that they can handle with facility and safety, and many ladies have discarded their old habit of frequenting our saloons.

2. Cécile Sorel, the actress.

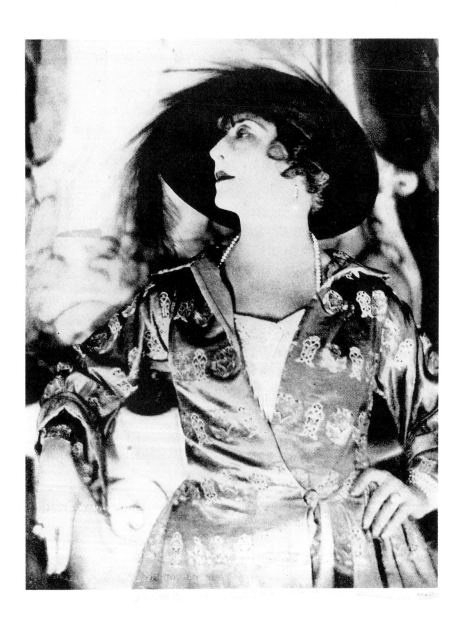

Figure 7. Cécile Sorel, star of the French theatre. From *Vanity Fair*, February 1921.

This fact may be explained thus: In the case of light fluffy coiffures, *i.e.*, the style requiring waves and curls – the aid and skill of the coiffeur are indispensable, but a lady can herself arrange a straight coiffure, either with her own hair or with false hair, which she can obtain from a retailer apart altogether from the professional hairdresser. And when she purchases her postiche elsewhere she also buys her perfumery there, as well as her hair ornaments, combs and all the other toilet accessories which the coiffeur supplied when the lady was forced to patronise him.

However, thanks to the sound reasoning and the disinterested counsel of old Trade workers – who several times have suffered in like manner in the course of their long careers – and thanks also to the vigorous campaigns carried on by the Trade papers, the Parisian coiffeurs have now come together in order to unite their efforts and amalgamate their best ideas; and they have understood that some pecuniary sacrifice would be necessary if they were to procure that indispensable arm of commercial warfare – publicity. Now they have decided to undertake a collective movement, which, it is hoped, will give the best of results. The big advertisers in the fashion papers, who, by spending enormous sums every year, render the Trade a considerable and indisputable service, have promised their support to the movement.

In a referendum, which has just been tried for the first time with real success by the coiffeurs de dames of Paris, on the subject of the style of coiffure to be 'pushed' this winter, there has been an almost unanimous vote in favour of the low chignon, combined with locks of false hair for day wear, and curls on the neck for the evening. The majority have also voted for waving. Everyone in Paris has set to work with these outlines as a general basis and with a free hand as to detail. The whole Press will contain accounts of these new coiffures.

If these steps do not suffice, the coiffeurs de dames will have recourse to the propaganda fund of the Federation Nationale, which at the Masters' Congress on the 18th and 19th of September, was augmented by the sundries-men.

I may refer in conclusion to an extreme method of renovating the coiffure and attracting clients to our shops, which has been proposed by a large number of colleagues, some influential ones amongst their number. This consists in forcing into fashion hair cut short and curled. Such a course would not make the fashionable Parisiennes hostile, but might tend towards a prompt return to waving, long curls, and remunerative postiche.

November 1911: Hairdresser and Client in Disagreement

Everyone, according to his tastes, interests and personal point of view, stands by his own preference. This is why clients and hairdressers are perpetually in disagreement, one might almost say in conflict. There is only one single instance where the coiffeur can be in agreement with his customer, and that is when fashion affords him satisfaction by decreeing voluminous coiffures which require a good deal of postiche and extras of all kinds. That happens every 15 or 20 years, but does not last long, for Fashion is essentially of a versatile and varying nature. Besides it would be quite unfair for us to seek to have the advantage always on our side. It is one of the laws of nature that when one has ascended high enough he must descend.

At the present moment, fashion is clearly unfavourable to our profession and in consequence to the allied trades. Take as a case in point that of comb manufacturers. Having, along with ourselves, enjoyed a lengthy period of prosperity, and having increased in number a good deal, they see themselves at the present moment confronted with a crisis of such a character that their association in France would be disposed to pay into a common propaganda fund (with the hairdressers), about 50,000 francs (£2,000) for an advertising campaign, which would assist in raising the turnover of their businesses. Moreover, hair merchants would do the same, and others would follow suit. This is sufficient proof that the position of affairs is felt acutely.

Fashionable ladies are only wearing small headdresses at the present time – coiffures in which it is, unfortunately, difficult for us to place much postiche, etc. Ladies likewise prefer their coiffures to look simple; they reject any complication, because this would be no longer in keeping with the outline of their garments, and especially with the modern bearing and gait.

Several hairdressers have offered some resistance to this unfavourable state of affairs, and they have lost their clients in consequence. Such coiffeurs are generally masters of classic hairdressing, and are, of course, master posticheurs. Having met with defeat in this, the first round, they have realised that concessions must be made, and they have just given way on the first point – viz., they agree to small coiffures, which does not, however, detract from their elegance.

As for the second point – simplicity – that is another matter. To that, I believe, the classic coiffeurs will never consent. They think that this will destroy our profession. Are they right? Are they wrong? I am inclined to think they are wrong, and for the reason for that opinion I have only to look at what is happening amongst the 'modernists.' This struggle is of such a nature that it is necessary to classify the old and the new coiffeurs. The latter, who in all respects resemble the artist-painters, do not wish to know anything of the classic methods which have been elaborated with so much trouble and effort by generations and generations of hairdressers. They do their work anyhow, so long as they get the effect desired by the customer, who they do not seek to educate, but simply to satisfy in her most incongruous caprice, provided that brings in the shekels. These young people do not think of what to-morrow will bring forth; they do not seek to prepare the future of the Trade or to improve our industry, but only to make money at once – and they make it. They are the only people who really work, because independent of their own *clientèle* they get daily clients who cannot obtain satisfaction elsewhere.

It is to be hoped that by showing a disposition to make concessions, clients and coiffeurs will finish by coming to an amicable understanding.

December 1911: Coiffure with Curls on the Neck

Discouragement is discernible amongst several of the leading members of the Trade. Feeling themselves able no longer to withstand the demands of their *clientèle*, they now make and sell anything that their customers require – that is to say, all descriptions and forms of postiche – provided that at the end of the week they have a financial surplus.

On the other hand, I find amongst others some well-defined idea – a firm determination to follow a definite model and endeavour to make it popular. [Several prominent] houses are at the present time endeavouring to push the coiffure with two long curls extending on to the neck, but on one side only. In France we call these long falling curls, 'Anglaises,'[3] this being an abbreviation of 'boucles anglaises,' as they were called a hundred years ago. I need hardly say that these curls are false; they are seen only with low neck dresses for evening wear, as during the day the furs round the neck would make their adoption impossible.

In addition, I have noted two characteristics which have become general: (1) A circular ornament, and, for special occasions, plumes placed on the left side without regard for classical rules. The more strange and extravagant is the effect the more it is looked upon as *chic*. My experience has shown me that it is when a particular fashion is on the decline that it is improved and made more becoming, more practical, and therefore, more tolerable. Thus, the circular ornaments to which I have referred were very rudimentary at the commencement. That is no longer the case. The supplying of these ornaments by the metre is not left now to the manufacturers of belts, ties,

3. Corkscrew curls.

braces and garters; specialists have sprung into existence who design and manufacture the ornaments with the aid of the embroiderers and jewellers, etc. As for the plumes, many kinds are made and sold at all prices, from those of spun glass, costing two or three shillings, up to aigrettes, which are sold for as much as 2,000 francs (£80).

3

1912

January 1912: The Wearing of Plume

In the face of the universal increase in cost of all commodities and the excessive degree to which the *grandes modistes* have raised the charges for their millinery, many ladies have reduced the quantity of their purchases; instead of four hats per season they order only four per year, and entrust the trimming of their out-of-date headgear to the smaller firms, who 'rejuvenate' them at a small fee. Business could proceed perfectly well like this if the leading milliners had not to pay a hundred thousand francs in rent every year and general expenses of proportionate extent. But their suppliers, who are at the same time their sleeping partners, cannot acquiesce in the loss of income which this economising process involves. Therefore, like the hairdressers, the *grandes modistes* have met together in conference, in order if possible, to arrive at the best means of creating business and saving their industry. The attendance was a numerous one, for all the modistes want to be '*grandes*' modistes. Amongst the most noteworthy propositions submitted was one which consisted of taking from the hairdresser ornaments and accessories for the coiffure, perfecting them and selling them at a high profit. For the verb 'to perfect' the modistes no doubt read 'to amplify,' for in a few days after this memorable meeting one could see at the theatres, in the leading boulevards, a multitude of fashionable Parisiennes, their heads covered with a sort of feathered hood, which would turn the last of the Redskins green with jealousy!

This struggle [between modistes and coiffeurs] had its *denouement* in the famous Revue des X . . ., a play written by several good dramatists for a fashionable theatre. The hairdressers approached the actresses who were engaged in this sensational Revue and not only asked to be permitted to dress their hair, but requested them to accept only ornaments for the head which would not conceal their coiffures. On their side the modistes also approached the actresses, pleading eloquently in favour of their industry, and offering to supply gratuitously the finest feathers ever found on the rarest birds. The embarrassed actresses, who wished to displease neither the coiffeurs nor the modistes, and in their hearts were delighted to obtain gratuitously all these usually expensive accessories, solved the difficulty by adopting a compromise which offended nobody, but which did not achieve the desired object. As each of them had to play several *roles* in the same Revue it was agreed that they should appear on the stage sometimes with the headdresses and ornaments of the coiffeurs, and sometimes with the bonnets and plumes of the modistes.

I hear that since that evening, the ladies visiting the theatres have been wearing feathers of various shapes and sometimes of very voluminous extent, and as annoying in their view-obscuring qualities as hats.

Of course, the illustrated papers of Paris are reproducing this orgie of plumes, and so ladies will not be afraid to purchase. I dare not mention the price, but let me say they are 'very dear'; to be in the new fashion with the ornament, ladies must economise in the price of an elegant coiffure. Once more, therefore, the coiffeur is beaten. It only remains for him to sell ornaments with feathers if he can, for the less pretentious drapery establishments, who, like ourselves, are up to date in supplying things to meet the public taste, can be relied upon to make this fashion common by offering plumes which are cheap, and theatre bonnets of all kinds. People now are going to the extreme of covering the hair entirely, and so dispensing altogether with the services of the specialist coiffeur. Nevertheless, we ourselves must rejoice, for the more this craze is exaggerated the quicker the ladies will tire of the monotony of such an unsightly and unsuitable mode.

February 1912: The Coiffure in Paris

At a time when business is at a standstill, the natural inclination, of course, is to devise some means by which greater commercial activity may be generated and some financial improvement effected. This is the attitude of many hairdressers just now, when after experiencing periods of prosperity, they find their profession passing through a kind of crisis. The position is solely of their own making – the result of an obstinate resistance to the inevitable course of evolution. Fashion at times demands certain concessions from hairdressers towards the wishes of their lady clients and even though in acceding to those demands their income may be less, temporarily, compared with more prosperous periods, yet they can continue their work in the reasonable expectancy of better times.

What has been done by those who have discovered that their commercial interests have been injured – and these form the great bulk? A number of meetings have been held at which their doleful plight has been related, and they have taken counsel together with regard to the best collective means by which the ill effects of the present unfavourable fashion might be counteracted. They have devised no better course of action than to form themselves into an association, invite the aid of other organisations and then inaugurate an artistic committee, which has in turn decreed an 'official' form of hairdressing to be followed and scrupulously respected by all coiffeurs.

It would appear that for this federated propaganda, there is to be a big financial expenditure in order to popularise this form of coiffure. So far, however, progress has been slow – very slow – as is everything which is regulated administratively, and all the time Fashion, in her unstable and ephemeral way, continues to change. She appears, passes, and soon disappears. What is essential is that she shall be seized at the moment of her appearance.

Being of a curious nature, I wished to discover if the principal figures in this movement – that is to say, those persons who constituted the Fashion Committee – had applied the decisions of that committee to their own individual establishments. So I visited them successively, and found that in not a single instance had this been done, which substantiated the doubts I had myself felt on the point. All these hairdressers are exhibiting very pretty models, but they do not resemble or conform to the style which the committee wishes to impose on the bulk of their colleagues. What is one forced to think, then, of the convictions of these would-be leaders, who themselves from the outset violate discipline and transgress their own decisions?

Now I return to the subject I left temporarily at the beginning of this article – that is to say, the example of the few young coiffeurs who are working and earning money because they consent to dress the lady's hair as she herself desires that it shall be dressed. Of course, they are not numerous, and as they do not proceed according to our own classical methods, they are therefore very much criticised by the other coiffeurs. But, nevertheless, they are producing head-dresses which please.

March 1912: The New Coiffure is Being Well Received by the Public But Not by the Hairdressers

My readers will remember that in last month's *Supplement* I concluded my article by stating that the Parisian waver, M. François, was the responsible creator of the new head-dress. This statement brought me several letters asking for further information, and the fashionable young ladies themselves are so troubled about this character of coiffure that they are constantly conversing about it with their own coiffeurs and even have recourse to M. François whenever they can find him disengaged.

In the face of this situation several of our young colleagues have commenced to copy this style of dressing' others pass and repass the shop window of M. François, making furtive sketches; and some would appear to be unable to get any sleep because of their strong emotions of envy and spite.

Everyone in the Trade criticised the new coiffure without knowing much about it, and so I thought it my duty to endeavour to calm the general disquietude, which was growing as the number of clients of M. François increased – or those who were partisans of his methods. Consequently, I persuaded M. François to give a public demonstration himself of his coiffure during the course of the last soiree of the *Capilartiste*. Before a large attendance and for a certain consideration, M. François executed his two principal coiffures [the 'Driane' and the 'Casque Oblique.']

Whilst M. François was executing his coiffures I heard some sharp criticism of this style of dressing, which is destitute of knots, curls, interlacings, and all kinds of detail. Numerous were those who found the headdresses lacking in prettiness, not practical or becoming, and, above all, unprofessional. They likened the coiffures to a Dervish's bonnet, a bundle of hay, and so on. Although I may be frankly hostile to this fashion, I nevertheless reply that the first coiffure is not buried away completely in the toques which the ladies are particularly fond of this winter. As for the second headdress, it is very becoming under those large and almost flat hats which fashionable ladies are wearing a little tilted to the right side. Moreover, these coiffures are likely to reconcile ladies to waving, and what is more important, the ladies themselves like the coiffure.

If the Trade thinks it must wage war against this headdress it will be of no use to criticise and show spite, for that attitude will not avail. More effectual will be the plan of dressing a lot of these models displaying them in our shop windows and on ladies' heads. When the fashionable folk perceive that their hair is being dressed like a 'hen without a tail' they will not be slow to adopt another fashion. Then will come our opportunity, for no matter what may happen, we can never find ourselves in a worse state.

May 1912: The Evolution of Fashion in Hair

When two interests are opposed to each other, the struggle may last for a long time, and even become continuous; but when several interests are in mutual conflict, generally it can be anticipated that the struggle will not be prolonged, even though it may be severe.

That is what is happening in regard to hairdressing. So long as the trouble

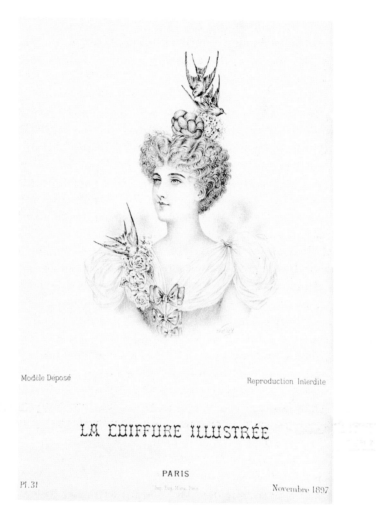

Modèle Déposé

Reproduction Interdite

LA COIFFURE ILLUSTRÉE

PARIS

Pl.31

Novembre 1897

Figure 8. A coiffure in the 'classical' style. From *La Coiffure Française Illustrée*, 1897.

existed only between the style of coiffure extolled by the coiffeurs and the fashion preferred by their clients, the end of the conflict could not be foreseen. Now, however, the situation is clearer, seeing that three distinct fashions have entered the field – namely: (1) that of the coiffeurs of the *École Classique*; (2) that of the clients; (3) that of the coiffeurs of the *École Moderne*, who recently separated from the others. It may be added that the last-named are marching forward with giant strides and gaining ground; they are making numerous converts and their number is increasing consistently. This arises, I believe, because they doggedly maintain one line of action and set a very clear and definite course, the opposite being the case with their *confrères* of the 'classic' school, who, whilst remaining faithful to their excellent method, yet champion individually very different models.

This lesson deserves to be borne in mind by those who care for their business, and particularly by those who incur great expenses by advertising in the papers. If we embarrass clients in their choice, and bewilder them with a multitude of different models, making it a matter of effort to discern the best, we shall not meet with the desired success. Exactly the same principle applies if we confine ourselves to proclaiming that we are the 'best hairdresser in the world' or the 'cleverest posticheur.' Clients reply that they hear the same claim on all sides, and that the mere statement does not suffice. When a big store is desirous of pushing the sale of a special article which it considers new and profitable to its business, it booms that article, although that does not prevent it keeping and selling other articles, and the purchaser is satisfied. Hairdressers must do the same, suggesting and indicating a particular style or model. Whether this style is perfect or susceptible to modification or improvement matters little – that will be seen afterwards. But, generally speaking, everything may be improved or modified, especially in the domain of Fashion – the most capricious and unstable of human fancies.

It is by these tactics that the coiffeurs of the modern school are capturing the public and doing the business. By pushing one style only, and persevering with it, they are gradually triumphing and leaving behind their colleagues of the classical school, who, although far better coiffeurs, without doubt, are too divided and undecided to succeed.

June 1912: The Return of Magnificent Combs

Without intending to recount the history of the comb throughout the ages, I may be permitted to recall that this small object of primordial usefulness, which lends itself so well to all the fancies of luxury and ornamentation, assumed at times, during the course of history, the strangest shapes and the most gigantic proportions.

In democratising all things the Republic has gradually caused [the most excessively luxurious combs] to disappear. During the great vogue of Marcel waving, quantities of combs were used, as I have shown in my Treatise on Waving, but principally they were practical models – that is to say simple and exceedingly cheap. The large quantities sold must have been profitable to the manufacturers (who had become very numerous on account of the demand), but it is now several years since the vogue slackened to such an extent as to lead people to believe that it was going to disappear completely. Some coiffures even do not necessitate combs at all.

Moved by this condition of affairs, both manufacturers and coiffeurs, for whom the comb is one of the most profitable adjuncts, have met in conference and, with the idea of averting disaster to this interesting industry, have compared ideas and brought out some attractive novelties.

By virtue of that eternal law which provides that every effort shall bear fruit, a movement is being promoted in favour of bringing the comb back to fashion. Not only are fashionable ladies beginning to wear the comb with low chignons, but certain indications foreshadow the return of the large models. Several of the great Parisian hairdressing establishments have exhibited some in their shop windows and in the coiffures shown on wax figures in the high-class quarters may be seen a good many of these large combs.

It is to be hoped that the coiffeur will be able to profit by this new introduction at once, before the drapery establishments take it up. The essential thing is to have pretty models, and both the select and to display them with taste and discretion.

August 1912: The Return of Powdered Coiffures

Now that the Paris season has terminated, and our fashionable clients have left for the sea or the mountains, we have leisure to recall that the three principal events of the first half of 1912 were: (1) the Russian ballets, with their agreeable features of art; (2) the Persian balls, given with great pomp by the last representatives of our upper ten,[1] which placed a lot of work in the way of our high-class coiffeurs, as well as artisans engaged in other trades; (3) the celebrated sale of pictures, engravings and works of art of the costumier Doucet. This sale was attended by the antiquaries and collectors of all countries of the world and realised something like thirteen million francs. As may be imagined, all interested in art, even those engaged in hairdressing, dressmaking and furnishing, were present at the Hotel des Ventes on this exceptional occasion in order to see this remarkable collection. The pictures and engravings of the eighteenth century excited extraordinary interest and unlimited admiration on account of their finesse and the prettiness of the young ladies they represented.

Two artistes in dressmaking, the Soeurs Ney, carrying on business in the Place Vendome, mediating over these engravings, wondered why the ladies of the eighteenth century appear to us prettier than those of the present day

1. The richest and most fashionable 10 per cent of the population.

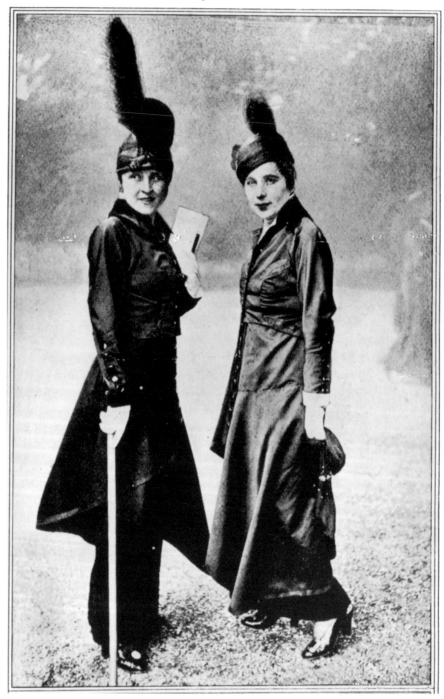

Figure 9. Fashionable ladies at the Longchamp racecourse. From *Vanity Fair*, July 1914.

and what could be their particular charm. They came to the conclusion that it all sprung from the powdered coiffure, and they at once decided to present their latest creations on mannequins with powdered hair.

This will explain why, at one of our recent race meetings, which all the most fashionable people attend, the gay Parisians were able to admire two superb young ladies with remarkable toilettes and not less remarkable light grey hair under their black hats. As they had young faces the astonishment was general, but everybody agreed that they looked very nice and, on the following day, all the papers announced this unforeseen event and commented favourably upon it. I noticed that several days later the English papers also referred to the episode. As I do not know what our London colleagues think of the matter, I am drawing their attention to the important fact that the master hairdressers of Paris have decided to push this fashion of powdered hair in order to bring about a radical change in hairdressing.

Like the Soeurs Ney, our group of hairdressers, in agreement with the Comité de Mode [Fashion Committee], has engaged two superb mannequins of twenty years of age, who will promenade at the races of Deauville-Trouville during the great August week, so that the newspapers may continue to supply the public with news of powdered headdresses.

This is the idea: Persuade the fashionable ladies to powder their hair at least twice; then, on the third occasion, explain that some false grey hair is much more practical and less messy than powder itself; and the object is accomplished! In the meantime, it is well to speak of the grey hair 'which is coming into fashion' and to mention it to every client. Seeing how numerous we hairdressers are, the advertisement will soon be complete and we shall not be slow to sell grey transformations.

I dwell on this word 'grey' because it must be understood between ourselves that we are not executing stylish coiffures and that we are not going to make our clients wear horrible, gigantic wigs of yak hair (like a Parisian coiffeur, with more ambition than talent, attempted last year), which have a ridiculously harsh and stiff appearance and the whiteness of which has reflections of blue, yellow or red.

The grey chosen for the modern coiffures is the pure grey of the Louis XVI period, a pretty light grey, but not a harsh white. Moreover the latter colour does not suit the face so well as grey.

Acting with the utmost disinterestedness for the well-being of our Trade, the high-class ladies' hairdressers of Paris, who are making great sacrifices of time and money, have decided to act impersonally – that is to say, act so that the public may remain ignorant as to where the movement originated. Each coiffeur, therefore, will proceed as he wishes and dress according to his own ideas, provided grey hair is to be found under the hat.

September 1912: Organising Fashion in Paris

There is every reason to anticipated that the 'important changes' in Fashion will take place in Paris, as has been announced already, during the month of October. At the time of writing, a great Parisian actress, the veritable guardian angel of Fashion, has gathered together in her Château de Normandie – one of the most sumptuous castles in France – a number of the best artisans in feminine coquetry. They include master hairdressers, dressmakers, comb manufacturers, jewellers, bootmakers, etc.

Handsome young ladies have been engaged on whom the new modes will be displayed; wax figures have been supplied for the hairdressers and dress models for the *grands couturiers*; and, lastly, the provision of every appliance and accessory necessary for the accomplishment of a complete and harmonious movement for the furtherance of fashion production has received the careful attention of the General Committee.

There is also in this château a professor of the École des Beaux-Arts, armed with numerous authentic documents of all description, which will be used in order to create discussion on the history of art and on which will be founded critical dissertations on feminine attire and decoration in past ages.

Thus it will be seen that the elaboration of fashion, which up till now has been regarded as futile, is proceeding on the most methodical and scientific lines.

Everything has been done with foresight. The meetings of these artists have been regulated like a veritable congress. On the first day (which will concern master-coiffeurs) the coiffures of the past will be examined very closely, and the representatives of the Trade will listen to the professor from the Beaux-Arts on this subject. During the second day, a study will be made of present-day coiffures, the nature of hats, combs and ornaments, and the methods which have been employed up till now to propagate fashion.

The third day will see the result of this work. At noon all the hairdressers will enter cubicles from which they will not emerge until three o'clock. During this period each must have executed a new coiffure on a living model and redressed it on a wax figure. At three o'clock all the models will go into the Hall of Fêtes where the figures will also be exhibited.

At five o'clock there will be a reception of all the fashionable and artistic people of Paris who are at present staying on the coast of Normandy. To each of the guests the Lady of the manor will present a voting paper, on which his or her selections are to be noted. The three coiffures which obtain the highest numbers of votes will be immediately photographed and sketched and then reproduced in ten engravings without the names of the coiffeurs who executed them being divulged. These engravings will afterwards be sent to all hairdressers who wish to be informed of the selected styles, in order that they may participate in the Salon de la Coiffure of which I have already spoken here, and which will be held in October.

October 1912: The 'Tie-Knot' as the Winter Novelty

The coiffeurs of my generation have already seen a good deal and had wide experience; but there are some other men who have lived longer and had greater experience. From time to time I like to have Trade talks with one of these, and show him our modern ideas, believing that in the course of his long career he must have seen something of a similar nature.

In fact, Fashion is perpetually repeating itself, and if it does not return in exactly the same form, at least one inspired to produce something which is derived from the past. Thanks to this practice of always looking backward and seeking out the genesis of what concerns us professionally, we can at one and the same time devise novelties for our clients and render homage to our Trade predecessors.

Powdered coiffures are now being much spoken of, but the question of powder concerns only the colour; before troubling about the colour it is necessary to know what the coiffure itself will be. Whatever we hairdressers do to amplify the volume of the head-dress our efforts certainly do not succeed quickly, for the fashionable Parisiennes continue to show preference for the very restrained styles. When the coiffeur obstinately insists on something else, directly against their wish, they leave him in favour of the waver, and then recommence the dressing of their own hair.

Starting on these lines, our posticheurs are at present manufacturing false head-dresses very soft and light, or just pieces of postiche, which satisfy clients. For the nape of the neck – since they have to simulate a pad-like chignon – they have contrived to make small torsades of very soft hair, resembling an ordinary well-rope, and their most fashionable clients are extremely delighted. A few also wear, as quite a novelty, postiche made up into a bow and, often with the tie at the bottom.

November 1912: The Winter Fashion

Ladies are always seeking to look prettier and more fashionable. To satisfy this craving they can never remain content with the charms and graces conferred by Nature, but must adopt the artificial aids of Fashion provided by the beauty specialists, the coiffeurs, modistes and dressmakers. This explains why ladies are always amiable in their attitude towards these people, and why they listen more attentively to the coiffeur than they do to the doctor.

But the hairdressers does not appear always to perceive the degree of confidence imposed in him by his clients; certain it is that he does not realise the commercial power which this blind confidence confers. For, if he were cognisant of it, he would bestir himself to profit by it, instead of losing the opportunity by wrangling with his *confrères*.

And if the ordinary hairdresser, without suspecting it, possesses this magic power, before which the most tightly held purses are opened when he knows how to make due use of it, what shall I say of the eminent hairdresser, the artist-coiffeur and the coiffeur-advertiser? They are really the masters of Fashion; they have only to speak and they are listened to and obeyed by the public, merely a gesture will cause the Trade as well as the public to follow them; in fact, they can play with their clients just like a cat plays with a mouse. Do they profit from this circumstance as they might do, or ought to do? No! They grasp their opportunity but partially; and imagine that they are benefiting a great deal. This means that they do not say the word, they do not make the gesture expected from them. They confine themselves to making many promises, but when the trustful clients come, they find nothing – not an idea or a novelty to satisfy their whims or to tempt them to spend their money.

Consequently, there are a large number of fashionable ladies who are fairly rich and willing to incur expenditure in order to obtain a new coiffure, a novel accessory for the hair, or an original idea in postiche, but as these things are not forthcoming at the hairdresser's they continue to take their money to the dressmakers and modistes, who are never found wanting.

The client, finding no new idea or helpful advice to be obtained from the man in whom she has placed her confidence, proceeds to formulate her own ideas, which of course, are framed on as economical lines as possible. This is why at the present time so many different coiffures are to be seen, so many badly placed plumes, and so many ornaments sold by the modistes or by the big drapery houses.

We have arrived at a point where the coiffeur no longer directs his own talents, but the client, on the contrary, furnishes him with ideas. The newspapers, too, instead of being able to place on record the creations of the master hairdressers, as was the case in former times, have to provide them with novelties. In these circumstances the *rôles* are reversed, and if this situation is to be continued, the prestige of the coiffeur must suffer and the confidence of clients rapidly diminish.

December 1912: A Parisian Eccentricity: The Pyramid Headdress

An old French proverb runs that 'He who wishes to tell an untruth has but to foretell the weather.' The fact is that even the cleverest astronomers find themselves deceived in the matter of predicting the elements, or see their calculations upset by a concatenation of unforeseen circumstances.

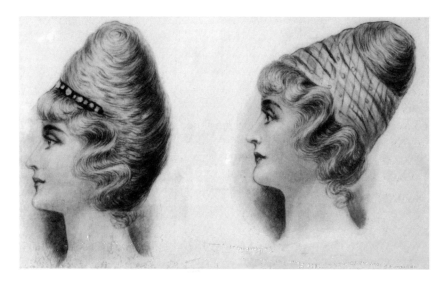

Figure 10. The 'Pyramid' Headdress. From *HWJS*, December 1912.

Exactly the same state of things exists in the realm of fashion and of things coquettish, although there the surprises may be greater and more numerous than elsewhere, for they are dependent on caprice, which finds a place in the character of every woman.

So long as the queens and empresses of France enjoyed the privilege of regulating Fashion as well as the affairs of the nation, the fashionable ladies turned anxious glances towards the Court, awaiting the gesture which indicated how they were to clothe themselves and dress their hair. But nowadays a host of little queens spring up from many different places, and in their turn hold sway.

The Arts, the Theatre, the world of Finance, and even the innumerable and toiling work-girls supply their leaders of fashion. That is the democratic *régime par excellence*. All those who conceive an idea possess the right of introducing it and have a chance of seeing it triumph.

For several months persons frequenting a large Parisian dressmaking establishment known for its eccentricities and enormous prices, noticed one of the beautiful young ladies who are only there to exhibit models of robes. The particular mannikin referred to was conspicuous as much by her plastic beauty, generously bedecked with several hundred thousand francs worth of diamonds, as by her luxuriant head of hair and the original way in which she disposed of it in the form of a pyramid. The news of her coiffure spread, and its originality incited much more interest in the firm than any other kind of advertising would have done. I wished myself to see her, and I had the opportunity of witnessing the lady dress her hair before commencing her day's duties. For, I should add, that when entering the establishment in the morning, these mannequins, like the actresses on arrival at their dressing rooms at the theatre, dress their hair in order to play the comedy.

Seeing that this coiffure was successful in arousing the curiosity of the clients who came to the firm, the other mannequins soon tried to imitate it, but were unsuccessful, on account of the difference which existed in the quality of their hair. They had recourse, therefore, to interior postiche and turbans of silk to sustain the edifice, but could never arrive at any other form [than that] which is grotesque. In short, the first coiffure continued to evoke curiosity, and gradually ladies have become so used to this original shape that some have tried to attend the theatre with something similar. They have not been quite successful, but as they are fashionable ladies it was noticed that they wore high coiffures, and it has been thought that hairdressing raised on top of the head will come into fashion again. See how simple it all is – no more than this is required to create a fashion!

One may draw the conclusion, therefore, that next spring ladies will return to a great extent to the high coiffure. In any case, we must not be surprised at it, and it would be well for us now to mature our plans with the view of profiting by this change and in order to abolish the front parting, which is the ruin of the coiffeur-posticheur. I do not think that I need dwell on the difficulty that we experience at the present time in getting clients to accept postiche for the front of the head – that is, postiche which accords with the dictates of Fashion and also with our professional interests.

4

January 1913: A Suggestion in Postiche from Paris

A renowned lady professor of music has just given in Paris her Grand Annual Soirée. In the programme, which was freely distributed, and even sent to hairdressers, there were the following items: Concert, musical interlude, ancient dances, and a public hairdressing competition; not one of those competitions at which the dressing is done in the hall, but a competition in the choice of coiffures recognised as the most attractive by a Committee of fashionable ladies and actresses.

Whilst the comedy was being played on the stage another little comedy was being very discreetly enacted in the hall. I was one of several coiffeurs there; each one of us had brought models with the secret hope of obtaining a prize. Man has his weaknesses, and the hairdresser is no exception to this law of nature. Every time that we met during the intervals we exchanged handshakes, each averring that he was there 'by the merest chance.' But as soon as we were dispersed in the hall one regarded the other with furtive and curious looks. Nobody knows how this famous competition of hair-dressing was originated – a competition of which each of us was thinking, but of which none spoke. For my part, I was thinking that the Committee would show themselves at the end of the piece, but up to the moment of the departure the Committee were not to be seen.

I began to think that this portion of the programme had been suppressed, by virtue of a clause printed at the bottom to the effect that 'the Management reserves the right of making alterations in the programme.'

Not at all; having passed the first door we found in the vestibule a few ladies who were kindly handing my model an envelope, and passing many compliments on her headdress. Of course, this coiffure was obtained entirely with postiche. The envelope in question mentioned: 'First Prize for Hair-dressing,' and contained a collection of picture postcards, as well a advertising matter from the donor. We left immediately, feeling rather confused, and I am unaware if my colleagues received prizes. I presume they did, firstly because their coiffures were very nice, and also because I learnt afterwards that all the envelopes distributed bore the same words as the one my model received, and had similar contents.

February 1913: The Coming of Small Hats and Their Influence on the Fashion in Hairdressing

We in Paris are now in the midst of the grand society receptions; balls, comedies in the *salon*, and dinners at which travesty headdresses are worn are numerous at the present time. In consequence of the events of this character some ladies are asking for Balkan coiffures,[1] others historical or fashionable and classical coiffures.

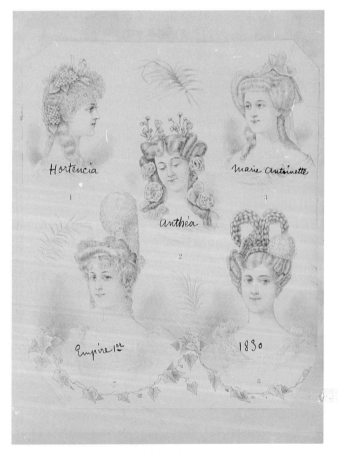

Figure 11. 'Travesties' Coiffures for Costume Balls. From La Coiffure Illustrée, *Album de Coiffures Travesties* (Paris: A. Lafontaine et fils, n.d.).

Ladies' hairdressers are at the moment much occupied in discovering what will be the future fashion in hairdressing. One thing has been clearly demonstrated – viz., that ladies are commencing to wear small hats and that this fashion will become general in the spring. Guided by this information, speculation is rife as to whether the chignons will remain at the nape of the neck, or be dressed on the top of the head – that is to say, within the interior of the small hats. In my opinion neither the one nor the other will occur. In saying this, I take into account that the hats are small not only at the edges but also at the crown. In these circumstances I think that ladies will suppress the chignon, perhaps they will even cut their hair in order to have a smaller quantity, and thus be able to wear miniature hats with very high feathers.

March 1913: The Eyes and Ears will not be seen This Season

Reassure yourselves, dear readers, that this is merely a cry of alarm, but as it has been printed by several Paris journals, I set myself to investigate it. And on looking round, I could understand why some persons persist in proclaiming that 'the eyes and ears will not be seen in 1913.'

Those who disport themselves in public places or parade the streets are not nervous or fearful about making people chatter and laugh. They are young ladies – not very elegant certainly, but very numerous – who exaggerate Fashion to the point of making it ridiculous. These eccentric people do not hesitate to wear their skirts so short as to exhibit half the length of their legs and a considerable portion of their stockings of golden lace, but they are very careful to hide three-quarters of their faces, which are elaborately made up. The first of these parisiennes has allowed her fringe to come so far forward, and has so advanced the waves on her cheeks, that it is in fact impossible to perceive her eyes and ears; the second obtains the same result by wearing a small hat, which quite envelops the head.

It is evident that if similar styles to these were to become popular, the ladies' hairdresser would have to close his shop; but fortunately, such freaks belong exclusively to a certain class of eccentric individuals, and that is all.

However, it has to be recognised that ladies are commencing to wear quite small hats. But these small shapes are rather favourable to our business, because they leave uncovered the whole of the left side and a large part of the back of the head-dress. Of course, the ornamentation of these new hats varies continuously, but the general shape seems to be fairly settled, being

1. The Balkan Wars were raging at this moment. Perhaps this inspired fashionable *parisiennes*.

altered very little by most of the good houses. There are some styles which are raised a little more, and posed on the right side of the head, after the style of the little Watteau hats, which were worn on the small powdered coiffures of the Louis XV period.

The ornamentation of the hat [shows that] aigrettes pointing in all directions are at the present time very much in fashion, in spite of the fact that they infringe all traditional rules observed up till now in the placing of similar ornaments. We live in a reign of irregularity, when the absence of symmetry is reputed to be supreme good taste. This coiffure is encircled by a scarf or piece of rich galloon from which spring the aigrettes; but often they spring from the hat itself, being inserted quite haphazard and allowed to protrude like the plumes of a savage.

April 1913: High Coiffures in Fashion

Since the closing months of 1912, very real efforts were being made in Paris to dethrone the parting, the bandeaux and the flat coiffures as being so many enemies of the coiffeur.

The Fashion Committee which has been formed amongst the Parisian ladies' hairdressers has at last been enabled to make itself heard by speaking to the public anonymously through the medium of a great illustrated society paper.

At the onset I should explain how this Fashion Committee has suddenly become a great force, notwithstanding that up to now the members of it could never agree amongst themselves, nor manage to persuade the newspapers to listen to them. Naturally the latter are somewhat like the Ministers. They always reply: First come to an understanding amongst yourselves, then we will examine your request. The Fashion Committee being composed of the classical and modern elements – that is to say, of coiffeur-posticheurs, enemies of waving, and of coiffeur-posticheurs, friends of waving – had to make concessions to each section of its members, and it was not until it had consented to these concessions that its true strength and authority were acquired.

Last month I presented to you the three coiffures which the Fashion Committee had arranged to be published in *Femina* in order to serve the interests of the coiffeur-wavers. You will notice that, as previously, these coiffures comprise combs and ornaments; that the hair is fluffy, but not waved flatly. I appreciate that there is a danger here for our profession, for without bringing any more money to some, this non-waved postiche may carry prejudice to some and incite clients to do their own hairdressing with their own hair, under which they stuff handfuls of old hair, which has fallen out, and often tulle and other material.

These are the latest coiffures published by the Fashion Committee of Paris in the great illustrated paper, *Femina*; all have been shown in brown hair, because blonde (and especially artificial blondes) are no longer in fashion. Hair in the shades of chatain [chestnut] to black is most appreciated, especially if it has a tinge of red. Henna is now the thing. Moreover, these coiffures have a very soft appearance, because they are made entirely of postiche. In this way, the posticheurs have mixed a good deal of short and medium hair with the long hair, making the coiffures appear so puffy.

May 1913: About Ornaments for the Hair

Woman's love for finery has existed in every age and in every country. The more civilised and cultured a woman becomes, the more she resembles the savage of the Pacific Islands in her taste for showy colours and glittering ornaments. If proof of this be required it has been provided during the past two or three years in our leading theatres, where all descriptions of feathers, placed so as to project in every direction, have been worn by the most fashionable ladies as ornaments for the hair. The forms of them may have varied a good deal, but their origin may in every case be traced to the coquettish instinct of the primitive and barbarous races.

If we examine ancient history we shall perceive that ram's horns, intermixed with very high ostrich plumes, were suggested by the blue wig of Cleopatra, the Egyptian. Floral crowns, garlands of foliage and devices made with precious materials were used in the coiffures of the ancient Greeks. Anadems, diadems and fillets of ribbon and metal adorned the headdresses of the fashionable Romans. The Middle Ages saw the use of *fraiseaux*, *fronteaux* (forms of bandeaux), coronets, golden hoops, strings of fine pearls, jewelled crowns, combs and pins made from precious metals – all worked in most artistic styles. Under Louis XV, natural flowers and ribbons of delicate tints were very much in vogue with white powdered coiffures. Then Marie Antoinette, under the reign of Louis XVI, encouraged a taste for ornamentation as well as for enormous coiffures; on the occasion of grand Court ceremonies each lady wore about ten ostrich plumes posed upright all round her high headdress, and an author of that period records that in the galleries of the Chateau de Versailles the vast collection of those feathers gave him the impression of a veritable wind-swept forest. Under the First Empire there was a return of the diadem combs, bands and plaques, finely cut in metal and richly set with precious stones, but of a sober kind, which pleased the taste of Napoleon I. Afterwards there were shell combs with large bulbs, of a shape and richness so far unheard of; these combs alternated with the return of the straw-binders and marabou plumes. Then came diamonds, spangled ornaments, bands of silk and leather, embroidered in light colours, encircling the coiffures; and, lastly, profusions of aigrettes, Paradise and other plumes of all sizes, *coifs* made of *toile d'or*, bathing bonnets, Oriental ornaments with turbans, small feathers, jewels and sparkling stones, pendants, small chains, etc. – all giving an air of perpetual fancy dress.

All this has now made way for something very different. In the quest for continuous change Dame Fashion has decreed that the exaggerated appearance of the overlapping clusters or clumps of feathers was unbecoming, being unwieldy and cumbrous. So they have been lessened in volume, and the exaggeration is now transferred to the height. Very attenuated and slender, these 'feelers,' which may be single or double, are shaped in the form of a note of interrogation. Loose flowers, stalks of flowers, etc., are also employed, and always of great height and fine and slender. Sometimes strings of false and hollow pearls, sprays of small roses, brilliants, etc., surround these ornaments, in honour of wireless telegraphy, and they look very comical on a small head and worn with flowing robes and high heels!

July 1912: Some New and Artistic Coiffures

I would certainly not think of assuming the rôle of theatrical critic, and before entering on the subject of this article, I will make just a few simple remarks. As in the case of most ladies' hairdressers, I have several actresses amongst my clientèle, and one of them has just played in a really extraordinary piece, which attracted the whole of fashionable Paris, because the charges for the orchestral stalls had been raised to a hundred francs (£4) each and also because the piece was advertised to run for only ten performances, although a million and a half francs had been spent on its production. It was called *La Pisanella*, by the great Italian poet G. d'Annunzio. Had I this gentleman's descriptive powers, I could astonish my colleagues by describing the fantastic figures and enumerating the riches displayed on the stage as well as in the decorations and the costumes. I will merely say that in this play, which is difficult to understand by reason of its very complicated and mysterious character, there were not fewer than two hundred artistes and members of the ballet. Of course, all the principal collaborators in this essentially Parisian play were foreigners, the majority Russians and Italians.

But that is of little importance. What does matter is that, thanks to our profession, I was able to be present at and witness this play, which numerous

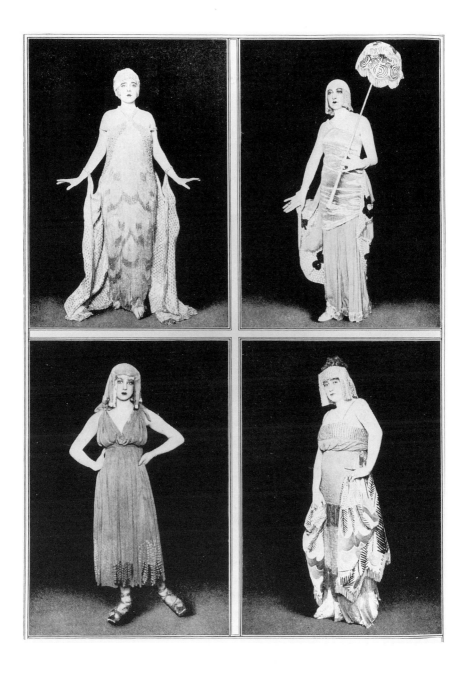

Figure 12. French Actresses in the Play, 'Aphrodite.' The costumes were designed by the great couturier, Paul Poiret. From *Vanity Fair*, June 1914.

wealthy people were unable to see for love or money. I am inclined to think that even at our prettiest gala representations of grand opera I have not seen such rich ornamentation of the coiffure. It is indeed a pity that drawing cannot adequately represent the array of dazzling diamonds which were exhibited in profusion in this Salle du Châtelet, where, as a rule, children's plays are performed. All the ladies seemed to rival each other in beauty and elegance. There was not one whose hair had not been dressed, and well dressed, by a skilful coiffeur. The general effect was excellent and inspiring.

It may be said that all fantasies are allowed at the moment. All sorts of picturesque comparisons presented themselves to the mind as one witnessed the fashionable spectators parading the corridors during the intervals. There was the suggestion of African palms, feather brooms, lightning conductors, greasy poles and bird roosts where parrots are replaced by flowers; one was reminded of antelope's horns, of lyres which are minus their strings, of marks of interrogation, and a host of other devices. They stand out in all directions, some straight, others obliquely in order to tickle the ears of neighbouring persons, or the bald pates of gentlemen behind, whose good manners prevent them from complaining.

August 1913: Coifs and Bonnets

Although it is always being criticised, Fashion was never, perhaps, so favourable towards the industry for the coiffeur-posticheur as it is at present.

What is necessary in order to stimulate a demand for hair? One thing only: that the hair at the forehead and temples is not drawn towards the back; that the new hair, or the 'roots,' are not uncovered. That is all. The coiffures may be large and straight instead of curled or waved – that is of no consequence; the means will always be found of dressing them, partially or completely, with false hair providing that the coiffures are of the kind that come forward on to the face.

That is what is happening at the present time. Consequently, we can earn money if we are ingenious. Independently of day and evening coiffures, which offer us a fine field of action, we have the modernised coiffure for the night, for sports and for bathing, over which coifs and bonnets are worn – nothing like those of former times, but, on the contrary, extremely attractive.

As in the majority of cases the effect of waving could not be resisted, it has been found quite simple and practical to place postiche around the face – that is to say, hair which will withstand rain, wind, perspiration, dust from the road and the dampness of the cold bath as well as the vapours of the hot bath. And, moreover, these postiches are not heavy to the head, because they are very light in themselves and buttoned either to the bonnet or coif instead of being pinned to the hair.

They can be dried when wet and washed in motor spirit after being exposed to the dusty road; they do not cost very much, since it is not necessary to match them very precisely, nor to make them up expensively. The hair need not be of the first quality; on the contrary, the more the hair is stiff, coarse, and dark, the more it has been affected by hair curlers and heated in the drying oven, the more chance there is of it giving satisfaction.

The small sketches accompanying this article [not included here] will convey an idea of the general shape of these postiches and the way in which they are used. They will also give an idea of the effect that is produced, even to the extent of making an undecided client purchase them. All these models have been seen or made by the person who is about to describe them. Most of them are furnished with fastenings or press buttons.

[The first] represents an arrangement suitable for night wear. As will be seen, from the rich lace bonnet, ornamented with small ribbons knotted into roses, hangs a fringe and some curls, which seem to spring naturally from the coiffure. But this sort of *négligé* effect, which men find so charming, is the result of long study and cost over three hundred francs. Apart from a few advertised lines, which they dispose of for 30 or 40 francs, all the bonnets of real lace sold by the leading Parisian coiffeurs cost several hundreds of francs.

The other illustrations represent bathing bonnets of various shapes and sizes, with the postiche that is hooked to them, and which is, as will be seen, extremely simple. Where is the coiffeur who could not make such postiche? All that is required is different qualities of hair artificially curled – that is to say, boiled for twelve hours and dried for twelve months near a very slow heating oven. Hair work of this description pleases clients and produces profit for the hairdresser.

In the words of the clever financier, strenuous brain work, but not necessarily hard manual labour is requisite if commercial success is to be secured. That signifies, in other words, that a good, original idea is often more productive than many hours of toil. My object in contributing this article will have been achieved if it proves the means of assisting my colleagues to add a little butter to their bread.

September 1913: The Coiffures of Parisian Modistes

Having devoted attention in this *Supplement* to the grand ladies of fashion, we may now deal with our less important clients – that is to say, those young

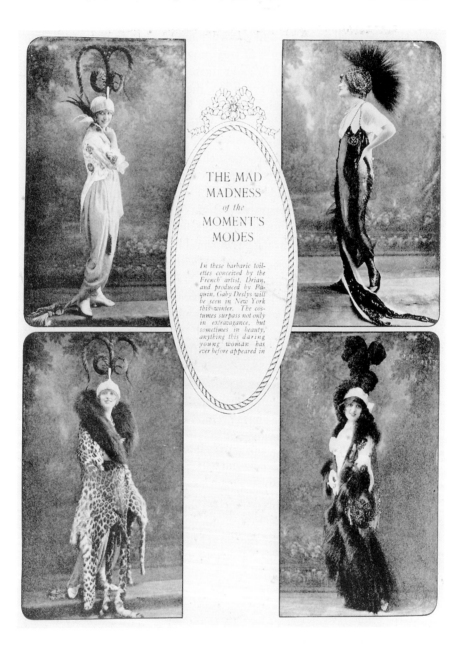

THE MAD
MADNESS
of the
MOMENT'S
MODES

*In these barbaric toil-
ettes conceived by the
French artist, Drian,
and produced by Pa-
quin, Gaby Deslys will
be seen in New York
this winter. The cos-
tumes surpass not only
in extravagance, but
sometimes in beauty,
anything this daring
young woman has
ever before appeared in*

Figure 13. 'The Madness of the Moment's Modes,' from the House of Paquin. From *Vanity Fair*, October 1913.

girls and women of the working class, who, whilst seeking to approach the styles *de luxe*, and being themselves frequently consulted on matters of fashion, yet have neither the time nor the means of imitating completely their more elegant sisters.

Ladies' hairdressers who are not married to modistes are not always well disposed towards them. They accuse members of the hat-making industry of ruining the profession of hairdressing by adversely influencing the wearing of postiche. However, nothing is farther from the truth. As a matter of fact, the modistes are slaves in two ways, and it would serve no good object of ours to form an alliance with them, because they can do nothing either for or against us. On the one hand, they are the slaves of the shape-makers, and on the other they have to bow to the whims of their clients. When the great and powerful associated shape-makers resolve to bring out a certain form of hat, which, for example, may be small and cover the head to the neck, and when in the space of a month the market is flooded with five or six millions of similarly shaped headgear, it is very necessary that they should be sold, and there remains for the modistes nothing but the variation of detail and trimming. As they can obtain only these small styles they have of necessity to re-sell what they have bought. And if a client presents herself with a mountain of postiche in the form of a coiffure, the modiste is compelled to make her understand that the fashionable small hats require less voluminous hairdressing.

But if the modistes are slaves to the styles of millinery that are sold to them or that they have to make according to the fashion of the moment, which is always influenced by the shape-makers, and if for this reason they can do nothing for us verbally, they can perhaps do something by way of example. We must not forget that modistes are almost as numerous as barbers. In Paris the barbers' shops do not number 3.000, whilst there are 2,500 millinery establishments, the lowliest of which employ at least two or three girls. In addition, there are others which employ 300 or more hands.

About those who are employed in the workshops I do not wish to speak; let them dress their hair how they like – that is of little importance. But I would draw the attention of my colleagues and the fashion committees of our Trade to the bad impression conveyed unintentionally by those modistes who come into contact with clients, such as the saleswomen and triers-on. The latter resort to a fashion which is most disastrous for our industry. [This coiffure] is what is seen everywhere by fashionable ladies to whom we are continually imparting the information that the high coiffure is becoming the mode. Three-fourths of Parisian modistes dress their hair in this fashion – and thus convey a bad example to the public. At least, this is what they say.

October 1913: The Latest Combs for the High Coiffure

I know it is not always easy to make young wavers understand that they must strive to sell postiche. There are some who have no desire to know anything about it, some even go so far as to dissuade their clients from wearing false hair, alleging that it makes them look old, is not hygienic, etc. They claim to be safeguarding the interests of their speciality, thinking that the more generally clients wear false hair the less waving will be called for. This is true to some extent. They think, also – those at any rate who wave for a shilling – that with postiche the clients can dress her own hair and has no need to visit hairdressing saloons. This, also, is true to some extent. The proprietors of saloons in which work is done cheaply need to have many clients in order to pay their way. But the people who run these saloons do not seem to see that if in addition to waving they prevailed upon their customers to purchase goods, there would be less need for them to work so much, and no ground for disquietude when their clients were depleted on account of bad weather or the effect of off seasons. Waving is certainly an excellent embellishment for ladies and an important branch of our Trade – but a branch only. Those who are content to make themselves the absolute slaves of this speciality may look forward to an unfortunate future.

However, the mistake must not be made of falling into excess in the other direction. A comb or a small piece of postiche are very easy to sell and also easy to place, whilst the large pieces, as for example the transformation and complete wig, necessitate special abilities which are not acquired except by long practice.

November 1913: Ornaments for the Hair

Hairdressers who imagine they can set the fashion or even think that they have the slightest influence over it are very much in error.

We are, my dear colleagues, the humble servants and even the docile playthings of this capricious and all-powerful fairy, but nothing more.

In reference to the subject of modistes and ladies' hats, as I have already explained, when the shape-makers have manufactured and placed on the market several millions of hats – that is to say, when there are no others to be bought – what can the modistes do against this wholesale invasion, this inundation of new shapes? Nothing, absolutely nothing but follow the movement. And willingly or compulsorily they do follow the fashions, which are sometimes favourable to them and sometimes unfavourable.

Coiffeurs do the same, and must continue so long as they will not unite and with common accord impose a fashion of their own conception. I do not think the day for this is near, although I hope and believe it will come, for hairdressers are great in number and will ultimately prove themselves very strong.

In the meantime, the fashion in ornaments for the hair is decided and controlled by the manufacturers and wholesale houses. These people resolve upon them dispassionately in their offices, far away from those whose lot it its to circulate them and farther still from those who have to tolerate them. The manufacturers (I do not refer to the manufacturers of ornaments, who, equally with ourselves, are slaves of Fashion, but the makers of fabrics, flowers, feathers, embroideries, etc., used in the making up of the season's ornaments) – those manufacturers are not embarrassed with our quarrels and are not disturbed by our differences of taste and opinion. They know that we are very numerous and consequently always at variance. They themselves are not very numerous, but they have extensive factories and heavy burdens to maintain; therefore they never dispute amongst themselves about decisions which seem to them of minor importance.

As with costumes so with millinery – the styles and material are decided in advance. This year it is pearls, next year it will be embroidery and another year it may be flowers. Once the decision is come to and agreed upon, it is brought to the notice of the large buyers and wholesale houses by means of a special publication called *Echo de l'Exportation*, and the host of small makers and shopkeepers like ourselves follow obediently – that is to say, purchase and re-sell what is presented to them, acclaiming it as 'the fashion.'

December 1913: Modern Millinery: The Hairdressers' Opportunity

After two years of immense hats, which almost entirely hid the face, the commencement of 1913 saw the return of small forms of millinery, and with them a small piece of hair was spread over the ears. As fine weather follows bad, so after the Trade stagnation occasioned by the bee-hive hats, hairdressers once again commenced to breathe and to hope that Fashion would be more kindly disposed towards them.

If we examine the most recent headdresses of the master-coiffeurs who claim in their advertisements that they are the 'kings of hairdressing, or of postiche, that they create the fashion,' etc., we may confidently affirm that their efforts (very laudable, maybe) have absolutely missed the mark. Fascinated by a *Comité de la Mode* which submits to the *Comité du Peigne* because the latter furnishes a good part of the supplies, the 'creators'[2] submissively obey the word of command, which is 'Let us dress high.' But with raised hats they ought to have dressed *wide*, and have created something attractive and novel in this way.

2. Long takes his models from the elite *maisons* of Lalanne (President of the Institut des Coiffeurs de Dames de France), Jourliac, and Heng.

5

1914

January 1914: Blue, Green, Red and Violet Hair in Demand in Paris

It need hardly be said that the leading hairdressing or rather postiche establishments of Paris rely, like the great dressmaking concerns, upon continuous and radical changes in Fashion in order that they may cover their enormous general expenses and even make a little profit.

Grouped together in the form of a Fashion Committee, the great Parisian coiffeurs have adopted the procedure of proposing that each season the change in hairdressing shall be a *radical one*, so that ladies may not be able to make use of the accessories of the previous season but be compelled to buy fresh ones. Still, it must be recognised that this stratagem, however ingenious it may be, is not always successful. Thus, two years ago it was proposed to cut ladies' hair and make it curl (or that curled postiche should be worn, which is the same thing). A few ladies were agreeable, but seeing the movement did not become general they abandoned it. Subsequently the Fashion Committee brought out white powdered coiffures, which met with but a poor reception. Last year (1913) from the beginning of October they caused mannequins to parade the theatres, dressed with false hair of blue, green, red, violet and other shades – that is to say, their hair matching the colour of their toilettes: their stockings, shoes, and even the make-up of their faces. The fashionable toilettes are now of these bright tints, called 'Bulgarian colours.'

The inauguration of this fashion coincided precisely with the revival of a play called 'Cléopatre,' wherein the principal personage wears blue hair, in accordance with the ancient Egyptian style, and it did not take the newspapers long to publish the news.

But is it pretty, is it befitting?

The dispute as to this point has lasted since the introduction of the fashion, and it does not seem as if it will finish. The last time that the bright-coloured mannequins presented themselves at the Opéra-Comique during a representation of 'Madame Butterfly,' the audience developed a touch of wry-neck through straining to get a view of them, and at the end of the representation the whole assembly was upstanding. Of course, the mannequins, although transported with delight, remained impassive, with the august serenity of priestesses of Fashion. The public were divided into two sections: on the one side there were those who laughed and ridiculed; on the other, those who found the latest vogue 'no more ridiculous than other things.' But the mannequins had fulfilled their mission, and during the whole of November the high-class posticheurs were busy making coloured false hair for clients whom they had been unable to persuade themselves, but whom certain dressmakers had sent to them.

The three pretty coiffures which illustrate this article were sketched at M. Antoine's, in the Rue Cambon. He was one of the first to use bright-coloured hair, and moreover is one of the most distinguished of modernists. To-day all hairdressers of Paris dealing in postiche are holding a stock of coloured hair and are doing business in it.

How Should this Fashion be Understood?

The newspapers continue to write about wigs, but we can easily leave them to dispute amongst themselves, for they know nothing about the subject. It is obvious that when a lady has to show herself at the Opera with a red coloured toilette and red hair, the coiffeur does not dye the hair this colour, and then on the morrow re-dye it blue. However, some ladies who would not wear false hair have powdered their own hair, either with coloured powders, or with powders of gold, silver or brilliants. Their hair is previously vaporised with water in which a little gum arabic has been dissolved, and the powder holds very well until the head is washed.

How Long Will It Last?

Nobody is in a position to reply to this question, but one may foresee that it will become general during the Carnival and then disappear next spring. If this be so, do not let us hesitate to make a little profit every time the occasion arises. If required, let us even create the occasion, for it is worth the trouble. Just think: A fashionable lady must possess as many postiches as she possesses dresses of different colours. That is to say, a single order may amount to twelve or fifteen pieces of postiche.

If I were asked why I anticipate that this fashion will die after the Carnival, I should reply that at that period we shall see the return of short and curled coiffures, and a lady wearing her hair dressed in this style would, if she had green hair, look like a salad which we in France call *chicorée frisée*.

February 1914: The Ears are now Being Uncovered

The changes of fashion are never very sudden or abrupt, but they are continual and must be very closely studied in order that their full bearing may be perceived. Mademoiselle Forzane, a young and delightful comedienne, who is attracting considerable attention in Paris on account of her elegance, raised her bandeaux slightly, thus exposing half of a very pretty aural appendage. But in order that the temples might not go free from embellishment – which would be considered ungraceful at the present time – she caused a nice little strand of hair to fall on to the cheeks. All the hair on the forehead was raised, with the exception of a lock similar to the one on the temples. This is why some fashionable young ladies are wearing in front of the ears – half or three-quarters exposed – a small strand of hair softly rolled or waved, with a similar lock on the forehead in place of the fringe. This fashion has not yet been adopted everywhere, and some folks are wondering whether it will ever become general. However, ladies' hairdressers should be conversant with this tendency, and ready to turn it to good account.

Like the majority of young ladies who frequent the high-class waving establishments, Mlle. Forzane does not wear postiche, except in the interior of the coiffure, as a support.

March 1914: Hairdressing Extravaganza

The Great drapery establishments of Paris are organised to compete with – and even to ruin – all small shopkeepers; also to injure the artistic industries by copying the fashionable models immediately they appear. The result is an almost general interference with business, coupled with no small amount of discouragement to the creative artists, who find themselves unable to procure any protection for their productions. It takes years in France to bring off a law action for infringement even when an article is duly patented.

Moreover, with their capital behind them, these great concerns will soon have no need to appropriate the models of others, for they are themselves beginning to employ the best of the well-known specialists. Under the circumstances the public could not be expected to pay exorbitant prices for goods they can obtain at cheaper rates, with a greater selection and more numerous facilities, since these stores give credit, take back goods, and so on.

The great dressmaking houses and the milliners, as well as hairdressers, suffer acutely from this state of things, which is becoming worse day by day. A lady purchasing from the stores a veil and ornament for her marriage receives gratuitously the attendance of a hairdresser to execute the nuptial head-dress and arrange the accessories. How can an independent hairdresser compete with such a system, which is a boon to people with limited means and economic tastes? One great store, in the hope of attracting ladies to its sales departments, has established a hairdressing saloon where attendance is given very cheaply by one of our leading hairdressers, whose fees are ten times as much in his own shop – one of the most renowned in Paris.

I will not refer again to the sale of postiche, which has a disastrous effect upon our industry. These establishments have for a long time now sold coloured postiche, and a large number of ladies' hairdressers are wondering still whether this fashion will catch on and whether they ought to start making wigs of various colours.

But I want now to refer to those who dress hair, and do it very well, without ever having been trained, and without being to the smallest extent hair-dressers. These people are more numerous than one might think, but we ought not to bear them any ill-will, for they do not take up the work with the idea of creating competition, but because in connection with modern hairdressing they have ideas which we don't not possess, and an audacity which the modern coiffeur will never have, seeing that he is imbued with his own particular methods and principles. Moreover, they have qualities which we lack entirely. They are mostly young designers, living continuously in the world of dressmakers, fitters and saleswomen, of modes and knick-knacks which interest the fashionable lady to the highest degree. They possess taste, too, and know the thousand and one things which, although nothing in themselves, count so much in the art of ornamentation. They exist in an atmosphere of feminine caprice; and are ever discussing and trying to demon-strate their modernist theories. They succeed because a lady likes to talk about these utilities; she likes to be presented with a new idea and so be different from others of her sex.

They do not make use of the iron or the comb; they do not possess, like ourselves, the science of finish, which hinders us in certain circumstances; but they can conceive a form and a general effect which we lack, emanating as it does from inherent taste and not from the Trade schools.

For a while some ladies have addicted themselves to hairdressing under these conditions. No longer selling many hats, the large millinery establish-ments are vending fancy ornaments for the head, and in order to dispose of them more easily they place the ornaments in the coiffure themselves, or rather, they re-dress the client's hair entirely according to their own ideas, so as to give the maximum of effect to the ornaments displayed. These coiffures are very extravagant, but certain ladies prefer this kind of hairdressing to the more classical work of the coiffeurs. There are young ladies at present time earning more money by improvising these coiffures at 20 francs apiece than they earned previously by selling hats.

April 1914: The Tendency of Fashion

The Front Entirely Raised

For some time past a number of fashionable ladies have been seen wearing their hair entirely raised on the forehead. This does not signify, however, that the fringe has fallen out of favour with everybody, but its departure may be considered as the commencement of its decline. As a matter of fact, ladies with low foreheads find the fringe somewhat in the way and are very glad to be relieved of it. Those who, on the contrary, have high foreheads, are ornamenting same with 'palms,' frizettes, fringes, bandeaux and 'low forehead' postiche. Ladies with medium-proportioned, well-made and flat foreheads are wearing slightly curled or wavy hair. Nevertheless, we must retain the new tendency towards upright dressing.

The Usefulness of Large 'Coquille' Combs

To offer sidecombs to ladies who dress their hair in the new style would be equivalent to offering them an umbrella in fine weather. There are some articles which cannot be sold, even with the greatest commercial skill, except when a need for them is felt. Large fancy pins are at the present moment selling very well, whilst difficulty is experienced in disposing of side combs. In such circumstances hairdressers should not be obstinate in their views, but rather offer for sale the articles that are demanded.

Return of Beauty Spots on the Face

Although this subject may be only of indirect interest it is none the less essential for hairdressers to know that the vogue of the *mouche*[1] has returned. The fashion is modified, as usual, in order to pass as a novelty amongst the young generation. In the 18th century these small rounds of taffeta and velvet were worn enormously, in different sizes and several shapes. Some represented a star, others a heart, a trefoil (club), a half-moon, etc. The great English perfumer, Eugene Rimmel, in his admirable work, '*The Book of Perfumes*,' gave the picture of a lady of the period whose visage was adorned with all sorts of these *mouches*, one of which represented a carriage and four horses at a gallop. The present-day *mouches* have this in particular: like evening

1. literally, the *fly*

wigs they are multi-coloured, and are sometimes painted on the skin. The position in which they are placed varies. Hairdressers who are also artistes in making-up have here an opportunity of increasing their incomes!

May 1914: High Coiffures and Crownless Hats

Ladies' hats are being worn very small – almost resembling men's headgear.

The edges, which ought logically to become larger and larger as we advance into the sunny season, are, on the contrary, getting smaller and smaller as if

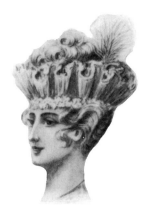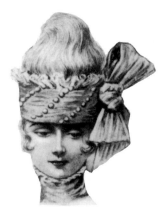

Figure 14. Crownless Hats. From *HWJS*, May 1914.

to defy logic; but such is fashion's decree. These very small hats are generally made with a crown of soft material, often of tulle illusion or net, and sometimes they are worn without a crown at all, when they resemble a garland or band. This form of headgear does not merit the name of hat any more than the flat headpieces which are being worn without crowns. However, we have to bow to this fashion, and to accept these caprices, whilst endeavouring to turn them to advantage. In this connection, crownless hats admirably serve the commercial interests of coiffeur-posticheurs, for the latter can build up and invent new and graceful coiffures. It is absolutely necessary that the top of the coiffure when it emerges from the hat (or rather the band) should have an artistic or, at least, an agreeable appearance. Regular readers will doubtless remember that in the issue of September, 1913, I wrote of the great wrong which was being done to members of our Trade by the milliners, who were selling hats which covered ladies' heads to the shoulders, thus rendering false hair useless. As if these modistes had heard my cry, they altered the shapes of their wares. First, the hats were made less deep, then turned up on the left side, raised at the back, and so on, until now we see hats without tops spread out into baskets and fitting as low as the eyebrows, as if specially designed to contain the bunches of curls which it may please hairdressers to build up and arrange in various ways.

In these modern temples of beauty and feminine elegance may be seen artists connected with all the professions *de luxe*, who take possession of a lady, divest her of her garments and reconstitute her into an entirely new being, so far as outward appearance goes, pandering to her tastes for coquetry and incidentally extracting all her available money. Nevertheless, she does not leave them with any feeling of resentment or regret; on the contrary, she is immensely satisfied. This is commercial cleverness!

It is generally the leading modern dressmakers who succeed in accomplishing this feat. They know how to procure the best artists for underclothing, lingerie, etc.; for ornamenting the face and head and the coiffure; and they gather in profit from this intelligent collaboration not only in money but also in glory and reputation. The most interesting clients rush into these establishments as if attracted by some irresistible force, not only because they know there are new ideas to be obtained there, but also because they are certain of finding new and exclusive materials of strange and sensational hues.

Let this serve as a lesson to hairdressers, most of whom are hostile to novelties and have a horror for initiative. Let the folly of the women and the audacity of the bolder shopkeepers serve as an encouragement to them to 'dare' to push novelties and to charge well for them. Fancy goods which really please have no fixed price; but they must not have been seen before. Let us empty our stocks and propose something new, and we shall be successful. The fashionable woman is like a doll; she must not be expected to have ideas.

June 1914: Is the Pyramid Headdress on the Decline?

All ladies, fortunately, are not foolish, but, nevertheless, how many of them cast aside all notion of good taste and commonsense by allowing themselves to proceed too far into the domain of coquetry!

Ridicule has often been heaped upon the styles of headdresses invented for Marie Antoinette by the illustrious Léonard. Those coiffures were admittedly rather voluminous and high, and sometimes ornamented with a certain amount of extravagance. Nevertheless, they were always designed in perfect harmony and were well-balanced. But have not certain modern coiffures surpassed in height as well as in extravagance those which were erected during the Louis XVI epoch?

Examine, for instance, the proportions of the coiffures illustrated in this article, notice their lopsided pyramid shape, leaning to the left, and ask yourself whether Léonard, being brought amongst us, would not in his turn be justified in making fun of the creations of our modern coiffeurs. Readers might imagine that these models have been submitted in order to cause astonishment or laughter. But this is not at all the case. They are, indeed, headdresses produced by the best coiffeurs of Paris and worn by those of our fashionable womenfolk who strive always to be 'up-to-date.'

Two years ago when I introduced readers to the famous postiche-enveloper which is used in the construction of these modern coiffures, and which stands almost alone to-day, I did not suspect that it would score such a success, or that it would be employed in the dressing of such strangely shaped coiffures. Much short, a fair quantity of medium, and very little long hair is required; fluffy, wavy and curly hair is necessary: a little of the last named but sufficient to permit of it running almost throughout the postiche. Hairdressers who have never handled such false hair, and especially those who may not have seen ladies comb it as though they were combing a sheepdog, cannot appreciate all the advantages it affords to those who have adopted it. With plumes shooting forth in all directions these models assume gigantic proportions.

It is hardly likely that coiffures of this kind will be long-lived. In any event, they cannot be made higher; firstly, because they come as a shock to good taste, and, secondly, because the majority of lady clients will not wear them.

Manufacturers of combs, and hair merchants, are very anxious that hairdressing styles should be of the large and high variety; they are incurring enormous expenditure in the way of advertising to push this fashion in the influential high class publications. But the public are clearly averse to this sort of headdress; the great majority of ladies are rightly in revolt against extremes, whether in the matter of costumes, hats or coiffures. And the hairdresser finds himself in the difficult position of having to withstand the influence of these different interests on the one hand, and on the other to continue to provide for his own livelihood.

July 1914: White and Powdered Coiffures

Our best clients will soon be leaving town for the fashionable seaside resorts, and before doing so they are making the usual necessary purchases from their shopkeepers.

As for ourselves, before awaiting the eve of their departure, and especially

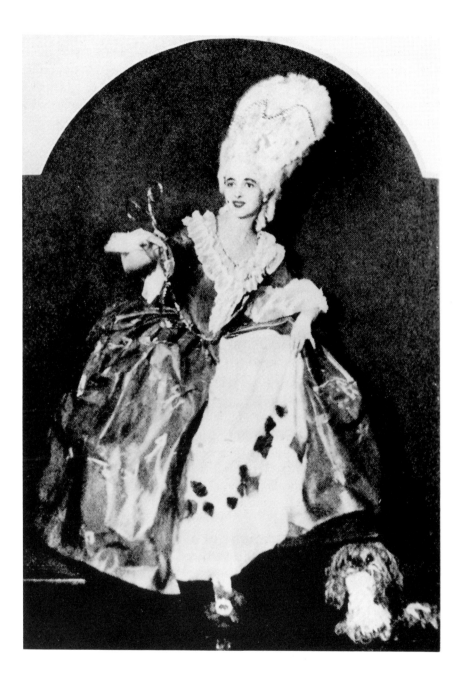

Figure 15. A Coiffure in the Style of Marie Antoinette. From *Vanity Fair*, June 1921.

before giving them the address of the 'best coiffeur' we must supply them with all possible articles, such as postiche, combs, ornaments, toilet accessories, perfumery, beauty preparations, etc. We must dye and wave their hair as much as possible and supply them with a special preparation to nourish the roots of their 'crowning glory'; also a small apparatus with which they can wave their own hair if necessary. Then when they are well supplied with all they require we may provide them with the address of the 'best coiffeur' in the place where they intend to recuperate.

Since we in Paris have had a Fashion Committee, composed of the master hairdressers, everything has progressed smoothly, for this Committee creates a fashion each season, and the rank and file of the Trade have only to follow suit and success is assured. Individually nobody can succeed, for no individual has enough power or prestige, or sympathy for his competitors to follow his example. If one individual proposed, or wished to impose, a certain fashion, others would immediately do the direct opposite, but a powerful group possesses enough strength to lead the whole Trade, which has willy-nilly to follow in its wake. Our one-time serious competitors, who were always fighting against each other, are to-day united by common interests and belong to this Fashion Committee. Thanks to this combination, every hairdresser may now overcome his clients instead of his competitors.

The Fashion Committee, after enabling us to have an excellent winter season with coloured wigs, will again furnish us with the means of making money this summer, for it has decided to push white wigs and powdered coiffures for evening wear. Already the daily papers are talking of white wigs. To some people postiche means wigs. And when a lady, having read the same information several times, decides to make enquiries in regard to these famous 'wigs,' and she is shown the little marvels of lightness embraced by our modern postiche-envelopers, she does not hesitate to adopt them.

August 1914: The Coiffures of our Leading Actresses of the Future

The National Conservancy of Music, Singing and Elocution, situated not far from the establishment of the writer of these lines, attracted special attention during the month of July on account of its annual examinations. The entrants this year included the sons of great composers and even the son of a late director of the Opera. Amongst the young ladies were several little prodigies in short skirts and with their hair flowing over their shoulders, who carried off the first prizes for their playing of the piano, the harp, etc.

One of my clients, who is a professor of singing, presented me with a card by which I was enabled to be present at these interesting competitions, and enjoy the harmony. But my chief occupation was to learn something about the headdresses of those who, by virtue of their successes, will be permitted this winter to make their *debut* in our first-class Parisian theatres, and thus become the queens of Fashion.

I must frankly confess that my hopes were not wholly realized. I did not limit myself merely to inspection; in fact, I was not backward in questioning these young people, and I ascertained for a certainty that those who possessed the most talent were precisely those who dressed their hair the worst. The only one who had arranged her tresses in the style so much in vogue amongst hairdressers at the present time did not win a prize, nor even a diploma by way of encouragement. Of course, the members of the jury could not enter into the question of fashion; they were all elderly gentlemen, whose own hair and beards left much to be desired. Moreover, they seemed to me to be far more occupied in listening to the music than in looking at the competitors.

The [first] young lady admitted that she had dressed her hair in three minutes. The [second] young lady dressed her hair [very simply]. She was not very rich according to her own confession, and could not afford to have her hair waved more than once a month, when it was done after shampooing; but as she played tennis a good deal she required a plain compact coiffure.

[The last] young lady is entirely opposed to having her hair waved with the iron. She has her hair shampooed, she said, every week, she carries out medical treatment for the scalp, and on the advice of the doctor refuses to allow her hair to be waved, so that she may always have a fine head of hair. I presume that medical gentleman in question is a very skilful advocate; I wish my colleagues in the Hairdressing Trade possessed, like this medical gentleman, persuasive eloquence in addition to professional aptitude. 'But,' the young lady added, 'in view of the present-day fashions, I should be far too ugly with all my hair smooth and straight so I attach under my bandeaux two false pieces of postiche for use when I go out – and only then.'

I had seen and heard enough; I retired thinking that hairdressers have yet much to accomplish if they desire not only to wave and make postiche, but also, and, above all, to educate all these coming 'stars' in the mysteries of coquetry and elegance.

September 1914: Hairdressing for Girls

In times of war, when everybody suffers more or less, the professions *de luxe* are, as it were, crippled, because other things besides personal adornment and coquetry have to be thought about. Coiffures and art postiche have temporarily vanished, like everything else which is not strictly a necessary. Those who ordinarily spend considerable sums in our business are now devoted to far more serious occupation; over their heads they may be seen wearing veils – a sign of mourning or of the functions which they have to fulfil in the ambulance corps and hospitals.

For those ladies' hairdressers who have not mobilised there remains just a little work of the hygienic order, such as the cleansing of heads and the making of small, indispensable pieces of postiche – work which is hardly of a remunerative character. They might also usefully devote their attention to the heads of infants and juveniles. Babies and young girls have not the same worries as we have in regard to the consequences of the frightful crisis in affairs through which we are now passing. They are as living and charming flowers, which give distraction and comfort to those who remain at home and encourage them to hope for better times. Their heads should not only receive great care from a hygienic standpoint, but also be well and tastefully arranged.

October 1914: Hairdressing for Girls

After cleansing the head, proper attention should be paid to the general effect of the hair. Nature has decreed that the finest head of hair (I do not say the

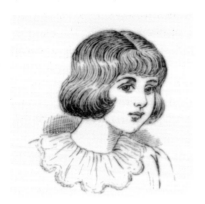 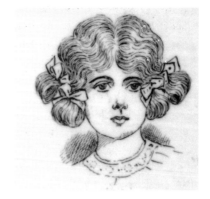

Figure 16. Young Girl's Hairstyle. From *HWJS*, September 1914.

longest) should be thick or puffy towards the middle, gradually becoming pointed at the ends. But it happens that fond parents, with the object of brightening up the hair of their children, make use of the scissors themselves, cutting off the hair in a single stroke, much the same as they would do if they were cutting of the tail of a horse. It is the hairdressers' duty, therefore, to establish anew the harmonious form [of the hair].

The essential point in our profession is the ability to achieve good results, to produce something pleasing and seductive. Some parents have a taste for the artistic, and would pay almost any price to see their little ones with nice, artistically executed coiffures; but a large number of hairdressers would not be capable, at any price, of executing a coiffure of this kind, because they do not believe it would be possible and because they have learnt how to do it. That is why I persist in this subject, exhorting young men who like their profession to practise and perfect themselves in this interesting department of their work.

November 1914: The Making of Dolls' Wigs

The European War continues with unabated severity, and until it ceases all industries, and especially business *de luxe*, will suffer from stagnation. Even from far off neutral countries – from the Argentine to Alaska – I am receiving letters from ladies' hairdressers complaining of the falling off of trade, and in some cases of the complete stoppage of work.

Until [the peace] those ladies' hairdressers who wish to make a living from their profession must put their pride in their pockets, lower their prices and resolutely attack the less pretentious tasks which were undertaken by their forefathers – namely, shampooing, dressing of plain coiffures, the making-up of combings, the manufacture of simple postiche, and the sale of cheap perfumery and toilet articles.

I have pointed out in recent [months] that a hairdresser who is not only a graceful artist, but also an ingenious workman and a resourceful salesman, should be in a position to create new business amongst his clients. I suggested, for example, how children's hairdressing offers a fresh field of operations, which should not be neglected, especially in war time. I now propose to draw attention to the art of making dolls' wigs, which is seldom undertaken in our profession. Up to now we have left it in the hands of other industrial workers to develop this branch, because we have had different and more important duties to discharge. But in these hard times we must take to the business and pay a certain amount of attention to it, for it is worth the trouble. Having attended to the needs of lady clients and their little daughters, hairdressers should contrive to manufacture some postiche for the family dolls, to take the place of the ugly old hempen and woollen wigs.

Hairdressers should explain that it is neither hygienic nor nice to place in the hands of babies dolls wearing hair cut from the bodies of animals – hair which can be neither combed nor washed and which does not lend itself to any form of coiffure. It takes from the little one half the pleasure to offer them dolls which can be dressed and undressed, but which cannot have their hair combed or dressed. Moreover, it has been observed that those children who possess dolls with real, long and soft hair train themselves, whilst playing with the brush and comb, to take greater care of their own hair. And the cost of providing a doll with real hair is not so very much, especially if ladies preserve their combings, etc. Such are the arguments which the hairdresser may advance in order to persuade the client to buy.

December 1914: Tableaux and Medallions: Hair Souvenirs

There is a custom which prevails in almost every family. I refer to the habit of preserving the first curls of a young child, and also the locks of hair of some dear departed or absent ones. These precious relics are always held in tender remembrance and serve to soften the sorrow which is felt at the loss of some beloved friend or relative.

But the members of the family circle do not always think of having the hair 'worked up,' and they are, even, unaware that these precious locks need preparation and care in order to preserve them from the ravages of marauding mites. Moreover, no artiste appears upon the scene to explain the matter and thus create a desire for seeing the hair assume a graceful form worthy of its rightful place of honour. And so it rests in disorder within some medallion, perhaps in some book; or, may be, it is allowed to deteriorate in the recesses of a drawer.

January 1915: Bracelets, Chains, Rings, etc., Made of Hair

Since the commencement of the war, that is to say from the time when modesty and simplicity took the place of the previous brilliant fashions, I have endeavored to publish a few ideas in the hope that they might prove profitable to my fellow hairdressers, whose businesses are naturally feeling the bad effects produced by current events.

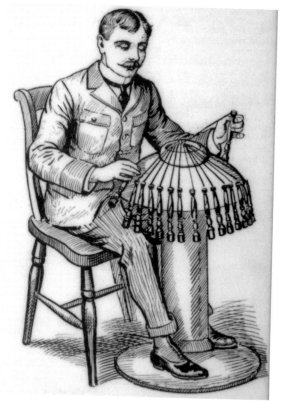

Figure 17. Contraption for Making Hair Souvenirs. From *HWJS*, February 1915.

It is now my intention to show readers how to make strings, chains and texture of hair, which may be worn in the form of bracelets, rings, medallions, tie pins, ear-rings, etc. This kind of work has been greatly neglected by hairdressers, and perhaps has also been a victim of circumstances. Still, those who follow my advice may find it helpful in counteracting the trade crisis occasioned by this terrible war.

What the Coiffeur Must Think of Saying to His Clients

In times of peace the weather generally forms the topic of conversation, but at the present time it is out of place to indulge in such small talk, and opinions are generally exchanged in regard to the latest news from the front. This gives the coiffeur an excellent chance of making a remark something to this effect: –

'Did you know that it has become the custom in Paris for people who are fond of one another to exchange locks of hair before parting?'

'–?–'

'– Yes, the men present the women with a small strand of hair, which is artistically worked up and then preserved inside a medallion. For their part the ladies offer the men who are about to leave for the front, or to visit some distant land, a bracelet, ring or neck band skilfully plaited with some of their longest hair. The custom brings good luck ... I have just seen (or I have just made) a wristlet for a watch, a chain of hair taking the place of the strap. It was quite an original piece of work. The mother, sister and wife (or *fiancée*) each supplied a little of their hair, and the chain, embracing several tints, constituted a nice souvenir, both elegant and precious. Here are a few of the various but more simple models.'

The coiffeur should now show what specimens he has. After the foregoing little conversation, the exhibition of the goods is particularly engaging and seldom fails to bear fruit. The idea is rapidly spread from mouth to mouth; orders arrive and require to be executed. There are specialists of this class of work, whom I do not seek to injure, but nevertheless I consider that every hairdresser should know at least the rudiments of this branch of the profession if only in order to develop it.

April 1915: Up-to-date Parisian Millinery

First of all, is there any new Fashion?

Yes! Notwithstanding its reputation for futility and instability, Fashion is infinitely stronger and more permanent than any of our institutions and sciences; in spite of all happenings and even of all cataclysms it survives

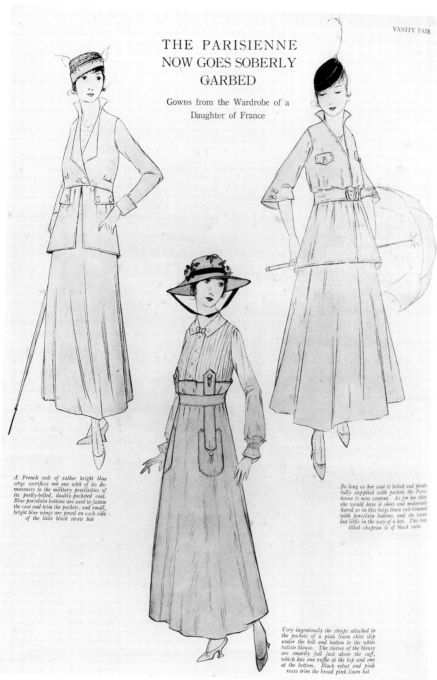

Figure 18. 'The Parisienne Now Goes Soberly Dressed.' From *Vanity Fair*, March 1915.

everything and everybody – Fashion is eternal.

Actuated quite naturally by current events, men and women in town present a somewhat military appearance. Ladies wear small coiffures, of the kind which cling closely to the head, and ample overcoats drawn in at the waist by a belt, similar to those which the soldiers wear. Gentlemen are again favouring beards and long hair, shorter trousers and closed jackets. Ladies are also wearing relatively short skirts, full corsets, taken in tightly at the waist, and high collars of all shapes, of which hairdressers must take special note, for the arrangement of the coiffure at the neck is influenced by them. Children, young girls, and even the little 'midinettes' [shop girls] don police bonnets of exactly the shape worn in the military camps, or else caps similar to those which are characteristic of the Scotch people.

These styles are sufficient for us to realise the kind of coiffure which is thus unfortunately forced upon us. The volume of the headdress must be restrained, as was formerly the case during a period of simplicity or mourning; waves soft and wide; little or no false hair; locks of hair hanging flatly over each other; the hair at the nape well fastened and flattened by the use of wide barrettes with bars; and a few light curls, coiled or slightly turned, suspended on the cheeks. There we have in a few words all we may hope for the moment.

This does not imply that ladies will no longer wear false hair; but we shall have to recommence making these accessories very light and practical in their character and use, if we wish to dispose of them as and when the shapes of the hats allow. In the course of time and ordinary evolution, larger forms of postiche will return also, but for the moment it is easy to see that the wavers will have more work than the posticheurs. With this new aftermath of waving, hair dyes and decolourations seem to be recalled to life again. The war is responsible for that. Hair dyes are prepared with ingredients which have become rare and consequently very costly. All fashionable ladies are profiting by this fact in order to brighten their hair. On the other hand, with the fashionable dark hats and also with the mourning veils, nothing is so pretty as a head of hair which has been brightened with a few warm-looking or golden colours. Those are coquettish sentiments which ladies would not care to admit, but which, if we are wise, we shall utilise to increase our professional business.

May 1915: Coiffures to Suit the Modern Millinery

Having fortified myself with the most reliable authorities – that is to say, having obtained my information from the highest sources, and my sketches from the best houses – I set forth last month the principal designs in ladies' hats which will be worn this summer.

As these designs are relatively narrow and go well on to the head, especially on the right side and at the back, it is not for the hairdresser, his clients, or for me, to endeavour to establish other forms of hairdressing than those which can be conveniently worn in connection with the hats in question.

If only we had to invent coiffures which were advantageous to us commercially, readers could absolutely rely upon me to design elaborate displays of false plaits and curls, with the addition of rich combs. Unfortunately, present-day circumstances do not allow of extravagant fashions or of voluminous coiffures.

Because they are not voluminous it does not follow that these modern coiffures must be ugly. Quite the contrary! Wide and soft waving, which comes more and more into vogue, permits competent wavers and posticheurs to decorate them tastefully. Then there are the numerous divisions with the comb and artistic dispositions of the locks of hair, which differentiate the work of the various categories of hairdressers and assure the success of the most skilful. It is not sufficient to wave a head of hair, or to cover it with a postiche-enveloper, and to comb the whole together in the form of a bowl or pyramid; coiffures of this type are not good and are far too numerous. The different movements of the locks of hair play as important a rôle in the embellishment of a coiffure as do harmonious waves in the decoration of the hair.

June 1915: The Vogue of Large Fan-shaped Barrettes

As a natural sequel to my article last month, I now present a few of the designs in large barrettes which are most in favour at the present time and which form almost the only ornament of the present-day lady's coiffure. We have seen by the models of headdresses published of late in the *Supplement*, and we know also by experience, that it has become much easier to sell combs than to place them in the modern coiffure. Whether small or large, combs are not befitting to the present fashion; if they can be conveniently used in connection with the hair they get in the way of the hat, and it simply comes to this: that the ladies buy without hardly ever wearing them. It is a very regrettable state of affairs, but it is so.

For a relatively recent invention, the barrette has advanced with giant strides, increasing and improving all the time. To-day it takes the place of knots or puffs made with ribbon or tulle, and the bunches of foliage, flowers or fruit which milliners formerly placed at the back of hats to ornament the nape of the neck. The barrette has become, so to speak, indispensable in all hairdressing executed without a chignon or with a raised chignon. Moreover, the output of these modern barrettes is considerable. Without counting the enormous quantities manufactured by the trade houses, there is quite an army of young ladies and real artistes of both sexes who pass their time in carving artistic barrettes out of hard woods, horn, ivory, mother-of-pearl and precious metals, either for private use or for jewellers. It is not uncommon to see these pieces of art figure in the salons d'exposition, where they are sold at several hundred francs each.

In the plainer models, which are more suitable for the hairdresser's business, some attractive shapes may be found, bearing evidence of good taste and a regard for perfection. Certain materials, which can be cheaply worked, permit of perfect imitations of the most costly shells, ivory, jet, etc. and contribute to the popularising of these small ornamental aids to coquetry and usefulness.

July 1915: The Fashion of the Large Side Comb

With the return of the fine weather, a first-class restaurant situated in the Bois de Boulogne, not far from the Jardin d'Acclimatation, has had the courage to re-open its doors. Those who are acquainted with the sumptuous nature of such an establishment will realise the enormous risk incurred; the extremely high prices charged render it accessible only to those blessed with wealth. Still, the restaurant in question did the right thing in reopening, and is doing business. There are intermediaries and industrials who are growing rich whilst the general public are growing poor; there are, also, some people who are so affluent that they need deny themselves nothing even whilst giving freely to relieve the distress of others. All such folk secrete themselves as much as possible in order to enjoy their comfortable circumstances in amiable company; and they are right in not spending to extreme limits – however useful that may be for trade – in face of the many who are suffering privations.

It is amongst the ladies who frequent this grand establishment, and also amongst those present in the boxes at the *fêtes* held in aid of benevolent institutions, that we are able to meet the finest examples of present-day fashions. Our remarks on this subject have been fairly numerous, and this comes once more to corroborate what we have already said – viz., that Fashion does not die, and even in the most doleful moments, amidst the greatest calamities affecting a large part of humanity, the other part does not abandon its aristocratic and fashionable habits, through the medium of which coiffeurs are amongst the first to find the opportunity of making profit.

First of all, the modern hats are worn slantingwise over the right eye, as we foresaw at the beginning of the season. This allows for the raising of them at the left side, and even behind, but especially at the side. The extent to which they are raised is governed by the degree of fashion in each case. The more *chic* the lady, the more care she takes of her hair, raising her hat to the left, and disclosing immaculate undulations, and the splendid jewels with which she ornaments her coiffure. The more simple, humble, or modest the lady, the more she covers her hair.

Whilst all ladies without exception are now wearing the large neck slide, the fashionable dames are also favouring jewels and combs of great value, which are generally seen on the portion of the head-dress left uncovered by the hat.

August 1915: Modern Millinery and Suitable Coiffures

One of our most intelligent *grandes dames* of the 18th century rightly said, when speaking of the feminine silhouette, that fashion sometimes gave in the form of a small bell and sometimes that of an umbrella.

At the present time the umbrella style has a tendency to disappear in order to make way for the bell-shape fashions. The most modern skirts are no

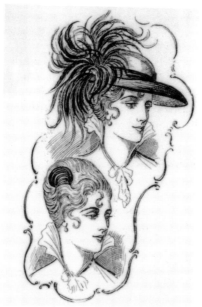

Figure 19. The 'Bersagliere,' After the Traditional Italian Hat. From *HWJS*, August 1915.

longer of the tight, hobble kind, but wide and short, so much so that some women in town seem to affect the dress of the Alpine skaters. This new fashion is born of the necessity of covering long distances on foot, as much as of the need of a radical change. It is graceful and infinitely more chaste.

It is a matter of congratulation also to be in a position to state that there is more restraint in general behaviour and less nonchalance in the dresses worn by the members of the gentle sex. We are becoming more reasonable and wiser, and it is not to be hoped that these happy transformations will not be exaggerated to-morrow by the fiends of fashion.

With the widening of the bottom of the skirt, we may hope, very shortly, to see the head – which is of particular interest to us – assuming more ample dimensions. Already the very small hats, fastened like bonnets, which reigned supreme at the commencement of the spring, are beginning to follow the example of the tight skirts and are disappearing; as the sun has become warmer, the ladies have been compelled to adopt pretty hats with wide brims.

[The 'latest' hat] is called the 'Bersagliere,' and our fashionable folk have adopted it since the Italian entry into the war. Placed sideways, with its trembling cock-plumes, the 'Bersagliere' is at once martial, befitting and graceful. Moreover, the 'Bersagliere' is the natural complement of the walking skirt, since it is habitually worn by soldiers, who are always indulging in this exercise.

September 1915: A Practical Specimen of a Coiffure with Chignon

One thing pretty certain is that the effect of the war will be to banish the excessive exaggerations of Fashion, which were approaching almost to folly. What extravagance of shape and proportions, for instance, the feminine head-dress had attained when the war suddenly brought us back to more moderate and wiser sentiments and more modest tastes.

Nevertheless, now that the war is being prolonged beyond all anticipation, exaggerations are being made in simplicity in the same way as previously they were made in eccentricity. Both have their defects, and incite irony or pity. Although the eye becomes accustomed to everything, it is nevertheless unnecessary, under the pretext of simplicity, for a lady to neglect her appearance and her good looks.

This is the line of thought which hairdressers should bring out in their conversations with clients, and in view of the great number of hairdressers there are, this advertisement, although gratuitous, will not be slow in bearing fruit – the more so as woman is, in general, very susceptible on the point of coquetry, and, whatever her physical trials or moral distress, she will never give way in this respect.

October 1915: Profitable Hairdressing

Since the Trade Schools of London, more fortunate than those of Paris, have been able to reopen, I take the liberty of making the suggestion that besides technical instruction a good deal of attention should be paid to commercial education, which will allow of dressing the hair on a profitable basis.

This question of commerce is of more importance than most people think. I have noticed, when inspecting the work of our schools, that in the majority of cases the question of commerce is confined to the selling of bottles of perfume, or other toilet articles. Obviously it is necessary to push all saleable preparations, articles and accessories; but I believe that before anything else, the coiffeur should pay particular attention to the sale of the kind of goods which have to be wrapped up in a parcel for use later on – at home. Anybody can sell them, and it is not absolutely necessary to have learnt hairdressing for that purpose.

The most interesting and lucrative article to sell is postiche – not the sort which is sold like a comb or any other addition to the coiffure, but that which is placed in position by oneself when dressing a lady's hair – to her satisfaction and in a way that proves the necessity of it. That is, moreover, what we should push, whatever may be the fashion of the moment, for there are more clients amongst those who wear postiche with discretion than amongst the smart, extravagant set who show it off with ostentation.

Examining the different styles of hats which will be worn this winter – illogical as winter hats appear in August – I have noticed that all the fashions have a decidedly masculine aspect; they comprise short 'top hats,' or the kind worn by postilions, Girondists,[1] dandies, and the natives of Brittany, but always discreetly and quietly trimmed.

As I have already had occasion to say, since the outbreak of the war, women generally seem compelled, either by economy or under a feeling of humility, to dress their hair in an extremely simple way – a simplicity in keeping even with negligence and ugliness. The more careful of them – those who patronise a good waver – have the appearance of [what] is, without doubt, a very graceful model, but the simplicity of which cannot last for ever. It is, therefore, our duty to combat this simplicity with persuasive arguments, and, at the same time to propose something which has more in it for ourselves.

1. The faction of moderate revolutionaries of 1792–1793.

7

1916

January 1916: The Work of the Trade Schools in Influencing Fashion

In spite of the difficulties created by this long war, some of the Trade schools of Paris have contrived to reorganise, and have even accomplished very creditable results. Amongst their number are the society schools, which are public, and others which are kept private, but which from time to time give public *séances*.

Since the beginning of hostilities women have been admitted everywhere, and they are particularly numerous. It was a young lady who scored the biggest success of the season at the competition of the Académie des Coiffeurs de France. The test set by Professor Nazaire was the following: 'A transformable modern coiffure: obtainable with postiche as well as with the model's own hair.'

If I may be allowed to criticise I should say that the undulations obtained with the irons on the natural hair were generally stiffer than the waves obtained by the water process on the false hair. Still, there are reasons and excuses for this. It should not be forgotten that it was, after all, a students' competition – that is to say, a competition of beginners who certainly evinced more earnestness and good intention than skill and experience. With such fondness for their Trade as they have already shown, there is no doubt these students will rapidly acquire the 'touch' necessary to impart a softer appearance to the waves.

Another original competition took place publicly after the series of classes so courageously undertaken by our famous École Parisienne de Coiffure, a glorious offspring of the Syndicat Ouvrier [the hairdressing workers' trade union]. The special competition did not take place between the students, but was an affair between the active professors of the school.

Impressed by an objection of the students – namely, that with the present-day fashions in low-fitting hats ladies dispense with the greater part of their false hair – the professors resolved to compete amongst themselves, and take the initiative in discovering a solution to the problem for the benefit of the Trade in general.

The young professors of the École Parisienne therefore courageously set to work, and now we have the excellent fruits of their efforts. One of them, M. Mandary, created a piece of postiche which he named 'La Croix de Genève,' [the 'Geneva Cross'] and which he dedicated to the ladies of the Red Cross. Different forms of coiffures may be executed by means of this postiche, from the flattest design to the loftiest. The demonstration which he gave publicly caused great enthusiasm.

February 1916: The Coiffure Changing Shape

It is often truly said that there is nothing new under the sun. It will be observed, however, that whilst drawing inspiration from the olden styles the artisans of fashion never copy them exactly, which may be attributed to the evolution of taste; on the other hand, they use their utmost endeavours to bring them up to date and in unison with modern ideas.

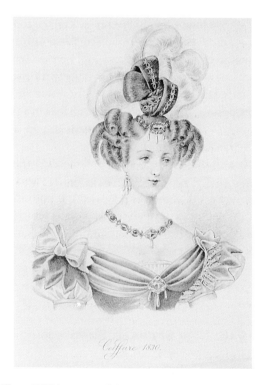

Figure 20. 'Coiffure 1830,' a new edition of an extravagant old style. From E. Nissy, *Album de Coiffures Historiques avec Déscriptions* (Paris: Albert Brunet, n.d.).

Therefore, by way of reply to the clumsy conceptions of our enemies, who, in their colossal ambition counted not only on appropriating the world's commerce, but also the sceptre of fashion, the Parisian dressmakers introduced in 1915 the 1830 style of dress, which met with an immediate and favourable reception.

What could the milliners and coiffeurs do when confronted with such a sudden revolution? They simply had to follow the general trend and adapt their creations accordingly. And the hairdressers being unable to bring out twice absolutely the same coiffures, unless the two occasions were a hundred years apart, followed the example of the dressmakers and the milliners; they modernised the 1830 style, whilst utilising the elements of present day tastes – namely Marcel waving, and the small characteristic comma-like or serpent-shaped curls falling from the hair on to the forehead or temples, in front of the ears and on to the nape of the neck.

We will examine the principal hairdressing models introduced to the public in place of the silhouette in the form of cocoanuts or Easter eggs – *i.e.*, the enveloping style of coiffure dating from 1910, which has now become distasteful, and which for all too long a period has prejudiced the commercial interests of our Trade. Our Trade leaders have realised the position, and, following the example of the great dressmakers and milliners of renown, have been busy devising some new creations. In conformity with their personal conception, or to satisfy the tastes of their clients, some of the big Parisian hairdressers are proposing an absolutely radical change in shape, whilst others are limiting themselves to such modifications as are sufficient to prove a preparatory measure to a definite change.

It will be seen that all these coiffures are well raised, attractively fashioned and quite distinct from the bowl-shaped coiffure. The variety is fairly extensive, so that fashionable folk can make a selection according to their own tastes. At present they seem to have no inclination to return to the light curls . . . the *ensemble* of which, however, is pleasing. The Parisiennes of 1916 have a marked preference for heavy locks of slightly curled hair, something of the heartbreaker style represented in the paintings of Spanish heads in the last century by Goya.

March 1916: New Styles of Hairdressing in Paris

Following closely the period of extreme simplicity in ladies' hairdressing, any new introductions that it is proposed to adopt will naturally at first convey an impression of extravagance.

In the creation of new styles two different sections are at work in our fashion committees. There is the group of 'moderates' who favour a coiffure of proportions which are relatively little developed, but which nevertheless embrace elements which are capable of profitable exploitation without startling the ladies with too sudden a change.

On the other hand, there is the daringly enterprising group who, desiring to bring about radical changes, proposed a 'grand sweep,' on the principle that 'in order to obtain a little it is necessary to ask for much.'

Amongst the leading Parisian hairdressers the moderate, cautious section, who model their ideas and methods on judgment and good taste, are nearly all established for themselves in suites of rooms; they have clientèles who appreciate their professional talent and are faithful to them, but who are added to with difficulty; whereas the other section, those who are more daring and enterprising, nearly all occupy shops with imposing frontages on the street, where they display, not the current fashions, but those which they wish to introduce purely for commercial ends.

Is this procedure a pleasing or practical one? It matters little. They only seek to attract the attention of the public and to fascinate them with fashions that are as showy and numerous as they are varied. It should be remembered that it is those who are the cleverest in disposing of postiche, etc., that achieve the best results.

April 1916: The New Headdress and the New Combs

It is very evident from the number of letters which reach me on the subject of the new style in ladies' hairdressing that the models designed and described in the preceding issue of the *Supplement* appear to be very bold in character, and even extravagant, to a certain number of hairdressers. This impression is really unfortunate, for in judging thus, according to their personal preferences, these good people seem to forget altogether the fact that in the commercial interests of all of us a radical change will have to be effected. And in order to bring this about it is absolutely necessary for the hairdresser himself to propose many novelties to his clients. Then it is for the public to make their individual choice according to their different ideas and preferences, and according to the financial means that they have at their disposal.

We professionals have a duty to ourselves, and it is for us to make up our minds that this radical change is going to turn out well for all of us. But between our own desires and the accomplishment of them there are always obstacles. The personal tastes of hairdressers themselves should not be an obstacle; it is rather our clients' ideas that count and are of importance, since it is they who pay, and therefore they reserve the right to choose what they please. With a sufficient degree of publicity, there will not be found many obstacles under this head.

There exists, unhappily, one obstacle that is very much more difficult to smooth away, and that is the terrible obstacle of the war. In creating such a number of grievously sad circumstances, the war cannot but foster the taste for simpler fashions, which very much retard the adoption of newer and more elaborate styles. The war has also deprived us of the services of many of our artists, and of numerous other material factors which are very necessary to give us all the publicity we need for the full realisation of our object.

However, the War, having commenced, will have to end some day; and it is whilst awaiting the happier times to come that it is the bounden duty of every one of us who is not actually fighting with the Army to fight at home in the cause of general economy, and for our own profession especially. It is necessary not only to know the Trade, but to be prepared to bring into it entirely fresh ideas and to aid in the introduction of new and profitable styles of hairdressing.

In Paris, in spite of the scarcity which exists everywhere, those who remain are doing all they possibly can, with the means at their disposal; all the shops are brightly lit and attractively equipped, the professional schools are being re-organised, and the hairdressers are all working in defined groups. The Institut des Coiffeurs des Dames de France is bringing out a publication.

May 1916: The New Coiffures and Hats as seen in Paris

The calling of a hairdresser is one that not only is pleasant and artistic, but also has a potency and an influence which are rarely suspected and consequently are hardly ever made use of. I am now referring to the way in which

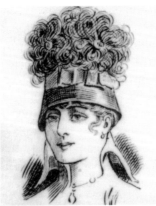

Figure 21. Among the High Coiffures of 1916. From *HWJS*, May 1916.

this calling can be made distinctly profitable. If only hairdressers realised what is within their reach they would all become richer men in a few years.

Nor would the hairdresser himself be alone in making these profits if he knew how to come to a decision; all the trades that follow in the wake – such as the making up of hair, the manufacture of pins, ornaments and combs, etc. – would be worked more closely in unison, with an exact knowledge of what ought to be done and what ought to be avoided.

Of course, clients always have faith in their own particular hairdresser, and frequently inquire of him as to the newest modes. 'What is going to be worn this season?' and 'What is there new for you to show me?' And the hairdresser often unthinkingly answers, 'Very nearly the same as we had before.'

This is a very big mistake on their part, for they should certainly have something fresh to impart regarding the coming productions in styles of coiffure, ornament, and in neglecting to show something new, something different, something quite novel, they are letting slip through their fingers very acceptable opportunities for making profits that may not come their way again. Almost every woman has a certain amount of money allotted for dress and adornment, and if the hairdresser does not get it, then somebody else will, for economise she won't and can't!

Amongst the objections urged against [today's] high coiffures, some of which are certainly very voluminous, is represented by the following query:

'How do you suppose that ladies can put on their hats with headdresses which are so elevated?'

Clearly, with the large coiffures which represent the fashion for 1916, ladies cannot continue to wear the very small hats which have been the vogue since the outbreak of the war. But a new fashion sweeps aside all old and established notions, and in order to accommodate the up-to-date high coiffures, the modistes have to-day introduced hats made with very high crowns, or without crowns at all, which permit of high chignons and loops and bows of tulle or ribbon entering the hat easily.

In short, ladies' millinery does not continue indefinitely. If it becomes necessary – that is to say, if the coiffures which hairdressers decide to create are unusually large – the modistes soon fall in with the new tendency, and the coming season will no doubt be noticeable for hats which are higher and more eccentric.

June 1916: Postiche for the New Style of Hairdressing

As was to have been expected with the present season's new designs in ladies' hairdressing, which are all very high, the postiche necessary for the production

wigs

of them takes a new flight, as it were, and has become distinctly more pleasing, as well as more profitable for the hairdresser. It is not only because it is larger and more ample that the new postiche is more lucrative, but rather because it is different from previous designs.

After the period of extreme simplicity, when the *industries de luxe* were, in a manner of speaking, ruined, the new fashion should please the public, and should, indeed, be very welcome to our lady clients. The hairdressers will design their creations on a more ample scale, and the postiche makers will produce work which is longer, thicker, and more elaborately worked. The mounts of the postiche will also have to be different, and it must not be forgotten that, with the longer strands of hair, the curls and waves will have to be in proportion, for this is one of the characteristics of the new mode.

It is apparent that these postiches are much larger than those that ladies have been wearing; in fact, they are more like semi-wigs, or even complete wigs. They are put on like a hat, after the natural hair has been rolled up on top of the head, or if there is only a small quantity of natural hair it can be twisted round the back of the neck to make a support; or, again, it can be divided into portions and disposed of, half on the crown and half on the back of the head.

In Paris all the up-to-date and enterprising master hairdressers are making these postiches and selling them at good prices, as something new. I should not like to venture on any statement as to the exact quantity, but I believe it is quite a fair number, because for some time several of the leading coiffeurs have completely stopped waving and are devoting their attention to the production of postiche, chiefly of this new style.

July 1916: How to Dress the New Coiffure with Several Pieces of Postiche

The fashion in hairdressing obtained by using several small pieces of postiche is interesting for many reasons; a large number of hairdressers find it practicable for many of their clients, and it can be utilised as a step towards more elaborate work; it permits of encouraging experiments; it lends itself to numerous modifications; and, lastly, it tests the professional ingenuity and inventiveness of the hairdresser, and gradually increases the expenditure of the client.

In order to sell the various accessories (postiche as well as combs and barrettes) it is necessary that the hairdresser should take the trouble to *dress* his clients' hair – not only to wave it and then leave the hair hanging down the back as is often done on the pretext of saving time.

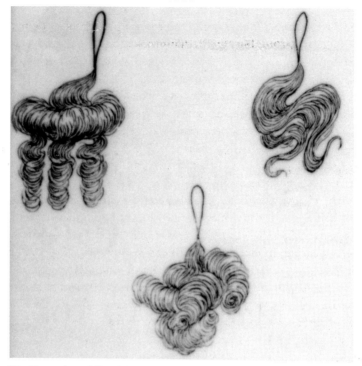

Figure 22. Examples of Postiches. From *HWJS*, August 1916.

I have in mind a striking example of the necessity of insisting upon this. An excellent waver whom I know, who had a good clientèle, continually complained that he could not effect any sales. At first I could not understand how this could be, but I see it now that he has departed for the season and left to me the task of attending to his Parisian clients. I dress the hair personally after waving, and am able to make very good sales, because during the course of the dressing I ascertain what are the wants of each particular lady.

To young hairdressers I will conclude with this word of advice: Dress your clients' hair yourself and never lose sight of the commercial side of your calling.

August 1916: Waving and Postiche as Adapted to the New Coiffure

Some Parisian hairdressers have gone to the front, and some to the watering places. Those clients who have not quitted Paris are patronising the remaining hairdressers, and some very interesting observations can be made.

No doubt, now that the hairdressers have left, the fair clients will begin to realise how much they appreciated them, albeit they tried their patience sorely at times. They do not, as a rule, want to change, for they realise that the dressing of a becoming coiffure is a delicate matter. In changing their coiffeur they have to take the risk of changing their particular style of hairdressing, for each operator has his own individual ways and methods. For this reason a coiffeur should always be very polite and attentive to a lady who is compelled to change her hairdresser for a time; and make every effort to understand just how she likes her hair dressed. A coiffeur who is alert can often learn something by examining the postiche of another hairdresser, and by listening to what the customer says he may be able to acquire useful hints.

Even if one has nothing much to learn, there is certainly little to be lost by being cheerful and pleasant; rather the contrary, for the client will then gradually forget her former coiffeur and any doubts she may at first entertain will soon change to a feeling of confidence, and she will be ready to take his advice as to the new wave, or the latest postiche, or different treatment of the hair, etc.

By the term 'treatment of the hair,' I do not mean only the keeping of it clean and hygienic, nor constant setting or singeing, but I include the periodical waving and curling (not forgetting the Marcel ondulation) which pay us rather better, and enable us more easily to dress the hair in the latest fashions.

September 1916: The Efforts of Parisian Hairdressers and Their Results

Now that we are in the off-season in Paris, it will not be amiss if we examine the efforts which the ladies' hairdressers here have put forth during the first half of 1916.

The needs of the clientèle (who had not been spending so much money since the outbreak of the war), and especially the change in the mode of hairdressing, have revived the work in those establishments that remain open. Admirably adapting themselves to the altered state of affairs, and practising in the industries *de luxe* the same unity of spirit that now exists in political circles, the leading members of all sections have gone forward hand in hand, creating new styles and helping each other. It can now be readily seen that confidence and credit are universal between not only the supply houses and the hairdressers, but also between the latter and their clients; and this improves business more and more.

But what is most remarkable and worthy of comment is the effort put forth by both male and female hairdressers during the past year. Each one has done everything that he or she can do to further the sale of some particular article, some novelty or speciality, either postiche, combs, perfumes, or other products for personal adornment. The small establishments in populous thoroughfares have taken up perfumery more generally, as they find it a profitable and attractive line; they are adding, too, a manicure department, in which they can effect further sales of specialities; and they are exploiting lucrative varieties of postiche for the newest fashion in hairdressing.

The more important businesses leave to them shampooing, waving, tinting, etc., and are devoting themselves exclusively to the production of new ideas in postiche, which are really most attractive and useful. Then, the big houses are selling more new combs – all real tortoise-shell – as well as dainty articles of perfumery, etc., very delicate and expensive. In their shop windows they show only the very latest creations in hair designs, which may sometimes seem rather extravagant. In the establishments of less prominence we find little ingenious introductions that are quite profitable, and useful all round.

October 1916: The Difference Between Ancient and Modern Hairdressing

Fashion may certainly be compared to a revolving wheel, but it does not necessarily follow that the models which are periodically recurring exactly resemble their predecessors. One is inspired by old styles, more or less, in the creation of new fashions, but there are so many modifications and changes introduced that in the end there remains only 'a something' that one might term 'after the style of a certain époque.' At the present time the newest coiffures have a little of the 1830 mode in their form, but that is all. They resemble them in no other respect whatever.

The principal characteristic of present-day ladies' hairdressing is its lightness and softness; the coiffures of the 1830 period were quite stiff and formal, even in the waved portions. All the old style coiffures had an appearance of hardness and rigidity, which is replaced in modern hairdressing by suppleness and irregularity. The universally adopted style of waving (in all forms) permits this advantageous change. Above all, tastes have altered entirely. Formerly it was necessary to stiffen the hair and support it with frames and wires, whereas in the present day we are continually drying the moisture from the hair to render it even more supple.

The symmetrical coques, rigid and brilliant, that were always seen formerly (which really more resembled coques of ribbon than of hair) are to-day replaced by curls that are very soft, and are mingled with natural looking waves that impart to the hair a state of perfect hygiene. It conveys the impression, in fact, that air circulates freely amongst the tresses, and that the dressing comb has no trouble in disentangling the hair. This is clearly an indication of a perfection of which we can indeed be proud, as wisdom tells us that we should follow as nearly as possible the laws of Nature, and Nature has never meant the hair to be left to adhere in one solid piece, but, on the contrary, allows for the greatest possible liberty and freedom.

The ladies' hats get higher and higher, almost resembling the old silk hats of gentlemen, and these allow for all sorts of fantasies in the hair composing the summit of the coiffure. These new curl postiches are very easily made by the professional, and meet with a ready sale at the present time. They arrange themselves perfectly in the large tam-o'-shanters which are now the rage, and are soft enough to take the thousand and one forms which caprice dictates.

November 1916: Fashions in Hairdressing, Ornaments, and Hats

The economists and the moralists are at present discussing in the daily papers of Paris nothing but the question of extravagance in the feminine toilet. This is an excellent sign. First of all, it proves that this extravagance really exists on a large scale; and if the indulgence in fashion and coquetry are again assuming such large proportions, it is an obvious indication that the grave preoccupations which have so filled our minds of late are disappearing, and also that money is becoming more plentiful, and is being spent more freely.

According to a critic, ladies' toilet goods and preparations form an enormous part of French exports, and constitute a sort of commercial monopoly which our enemies are trying desperately to wrest from us, on account of the immense number of workers to whom employment is given. Nevertheless, in the midst of the universal mourning which the war has occasioned, when no woman can help feeling depressed as she thinks of the peril that overhangs her loved one, ought Frenchwomen (who have the means) to think about coquetry and extravagance? Cruel dilemma! Public sentiment is scandalised. It seems out of place indeed, to think of luxury when one contemplates the number of wounded, and sees the soldiers on leave who have suffered so much on the battlefield. But then, on the other hand, there is the risk of depriving thousands of workers of their means of livelihood, and, moreover, the innate regard for coquetry remains unsatisfied.

One seems tempted to apply to this problem the phrase 'Use but don't abuse.' In other words, 'Continue your visits to your hairdresser and coiffeur, ladies, but in moderation.' Yes, but who is to draw the line and decide where

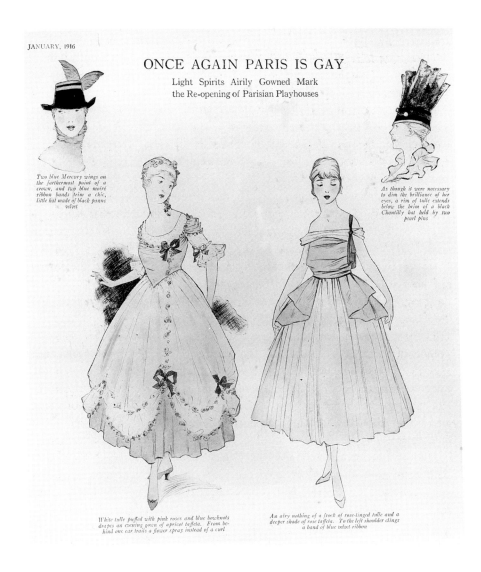

ONCE AGAIN PARIS IS GAY

Light Spirits Airily Gowned Mark
the Re-opening of Parisian Playhouses

Two blue Mercury wings on the farthermost point of a crown, and two blue moiré ribbon bands trim a chic, little hat made of black panne velvet

As though it were necessary to dim the brilliance of her eyes, a rim of tulle extends below the brim of a black Chantilly hat held by two pearl pins

White tulle puffed with pink roses and blue bowknots drapes an evening gown of apricot taffeta. From behind one ear trails a flower spray instead of a curl

An airy nothing of a frock of rose-tinged tulle and a deeper shade of rose taffeta. To the left shoulder clings a band of blue velvet ribbon

Figure 23. 'Once Again Paris is Gay.' From *Vanity Fair*, January 1916.

the term 'moderation' is to cease? Each lady will be tempted to establish her own point of view regarding this question. She will say to herself, 'Anything that I can pay for is reasonable; extravagance is the amount that is spent by persons richer than myself.' Ladies, in fact, are quite naturally inclined to apply the doctrine of equality to dress in the same way as each one of us exclaims: 'Equality! Yes, but with our superiors.' The most convincing writers and the severest critics are impotent before the eternal and essentially human regard for personal attraction, to the institution of which we owe even our profession.

Study a picture of a Parisienne dressed in the latest style for 1916, and you will be astonished at the mixture of eccentricity and audacity: coiffures extremely high, skirts excessively short, dresses decidedly décolleté, and faces inordinately painted. Everything has gone to the extreme, quite the opposite to the practice of a few seasons ago.

Of course, as will be understood, I am not referring to every Parisienne, but to the very large number of leaders of fashion who exhibit these gowns in the smart cafés, restaurants and tea-shops, and in any other rendezvous where they can create a sensation. Other women regard this ultra smart set first of all with curiosity, then with a certain feeling of pleasure, and finally they copy them more or less.

These are the latest characteristics. The coiffure is still dressed high, and even perhaps a little higher. The fashionable tint at the present is brunette – the classic tints of lilies and roses are no longer in vogue. The powders and creams of the moment give a colour almost as dark as a mulatto; the rouge is dark brick colour; eyelashes are violet, blue, and mauve. The ears are adorned with long green ear-rings, with necklaces to match.

The hands are made up quite as much as the face, nails being worn long and very red. The watch bracelet is replaced by an identification bracelet entirely in shell.

Hair ornaments are worn over the eyes, as are also the hats . . . The higher the hat the smarter the wearer. We cannot mention all the forms of extravagance, as too much space would be needed to enumerate them and above all to describe them.

December 1916: Coiffures and Ornaments de Luxe

The daily papers of Paris continue their discussions on the utility and expediency of luxury at the present time. The general theme seems to be 'Ought we to condemn or acquit those persons who are guilty of extravagant expenditure?'

Never, in fact, has the Press taken up this question so thoroughly, and yet they have not arrived at any definite conclusion on the subject. According to some the money that is spent on things that are not absolutely necessary could be used to better advantage. Others hold that the first necessity is to see that commerce does not come to a standstill whatever else happens, and at any rate the circulation of money assures that the workers are not out of employment.

As a matter of fact it is those who entertain the latter opinion who have the great majority of ladies on their side, for there are many of the fair sex who consider life would not be worth living if they could not follow the latest ideas in coquetry and fashion.

Meanwhile, while the papers put forward their points of view, all the industries progress and prosper. The ladies' coiffeurs create new models, the smart posticheurs can hardly find enough material to keep them going, the onduleurs are overworked, comb manufacturers are flooding the country with innumerable fantasies, and perfumers are for ever bringing out fresh novelties.

But we could do better still if the necessities of the war did not cause a large diminution in the supplies of materials and workers, if we were not compelled to close the workshops and stores so early in order to avoid expenditure of electricity and gas, and thus leave sufficient for the munition factories, which are in full swing day and night and get more numerous every day.

The first-class coiffeurs are continually creating new models. This can be seen by a walk though the principal arteries of our capital and taking note of the magnificent professional effort that is now being made. If we only look at the windows of the coiffeurs' and posticheurs' establishment, we shall notice this, but we must remember that all the members of our craft are not established in shops; the majority are to be found on the floors above – in flats that are practically private, because they are generally composed of a number of consecutive rooms, and although one can easily obtain admittance into the first one, it is very difficult to get any farther, as to reach the main ateliers it is necessary to show a 'patte blanche.' That is to say, one must either produce an introduction from a well-known house, or else be a well-known coiffeur oneself, as it is in these apartments that the master coiffeurs are at work on the newest modes, which are nearly always reserved for their best customers. The smart coiffeurs of Paris are, like the best dressmaking houses and milliners, aware of the competition which exists, and know that their most profitable productions are quickly copied and hundreds sold at bargain prices, if they are not kept carefully hidden.

Besides this, clients who are willing to pay a large sum for a new style wish to be to a certain extent the only wearers of it. And these models are really reserved for them. How many ladies have gone up these stairs in vain, even when they have been willing to pay no matter how much. Unnecessary journey! The drawers are not opened and the models are not shown if the person is not recommended or known by the firm. The lady receives the polite reply that the models are not yet ready – that is all. And each time the same thing happens. The latest novelties are never shown to persons of that category.

8

1917

January 1917: The Evolution of the Perfumery Business

By decreeing that in the interests of the State evening dress can no longer be worn in theatres, the Government have struck a heavy blow at hairdressers who make a speciality of fancy hairdressing. However, prevailing circumstances do not permit me to go further into the subject at the present time, and it must be postponed until a later date.

Another question of interest and importance at the moment is the recrudescence of activity amongst French chemists [i.e., pharmacies] in their attack on coiffeurs, perfumers and beauty specialists.

During the period intervening between the War of 1870 and the present War, the commerce in these products gradually extended until it attained almost incredible proportions. Indulgence in luxury increased beyond all bounds. Even coiffeurs de dames in a small way of business could easily dispose of cosmetics or perfumery costing 50 francs (£2) per box, and 100 francs (£4) for a small flagon. The flagons and boxes were made very artistically, often bore the signatures of renowned artistes, and were contained in dainty caskets that in turn were delicately enclosed in other protective coverings.

To-day, such articles are still exhibited in the windows of the best firms, but there is hardly any demand for them, and several of these caskets that I have seen offered for sale no longer bear their original beauty and freshness. The period of economy in France, voluntary or compulsory, has naturally revolutionised all businesses, including that of perfumery. But such commerce will never really cease; like our own profession and any other which ministers to coquetterie and elegance, it is permanent and continuous. [But] it arranges itself to suit the exigencies of the period, and awaits more propitious times.

Taking into consideration the necessities of the moment, those innovators who are willing to take risks have a good chance of succeeding at the present time. Amongst their many attempts, I will mention one that has caused quite a sensation, as much amongst the public as amongst hairdressers.

A young man – who, by the way, does not belong to our calling, but who does not lack in skill or originality – has established in the eccentric quarter of Montmartre an unpretentious shop that has been enlarged from time to time. He commenced by making a speciality of selling well-known perfumery and toilet articles by weight in small quantities. The shop was fitted up very plainly – a few deal shelves on each of the four walls, with a sort of grocer's counter, and a drawer beneath. The stock consisted of large bottles, containing various coloured liquids, and also large jars in which were toilet creams and powders.

In the front window were placed several broken jars, similar to those in which our own Trade goods are exhibited, with advertising matter a samples which were designed to demonstrate the advantages of the goods offered for sale over those produced by competing houses.

The shop was soon filled with customers. It was just as easy to obtain 10 grammes of any well-known perfume as it was to buy 10 grammes of any of the proprietor's own brands, only the latter were necessarily much cheaper. On the door a crowd read the following inscription: –

The Perfumery Business is a Business of Disguises. The Jar, the Casket, the Label and the Ribbon cost more than the Perfume itself. Here we sell by Weight and not by Appearance, therefore our Customers only pay for what they really obtain. You will be supplied in your own jar with any quantity of any well-known brand that you desire. The Perfumes are priced at so much per gramme.

After a little time, certain of the proprietors of these 'well-known' lines, on account of their retail customers' complaints, took steps to prevent this traffic in their best selling goods. Then the 'well-known' brands of perfumes disappeared discreetly from the counter, but not from the advertisements and catalogues. But the unbranded perfumes, without label or casket, sold very well. The public had already got used to them; the picturesque inscriptions with their Parisian slang greatly augmented the advertisement. Now the shop has been enlarged, and is more luxuriously fitted. Having tried perfumery, other goods are being exploited, to the detriment of the hairdressers' sale trade. A sign six yards long displayed on the front of the shop announces:

Manicure, 75 centimes (7½d.), and it is worth no more.

Result, a further enlargement of premises. And now a ladies' hairdressing saloon has succeeded equally well. Clients are waited upon by lady assistants, and there is always a crowd of customers seeking admittance.

February 1917: Ladies' Hairdressing at the Paris Academies

This terrible war has changed many things to which we were accustomed. For example, previously we thought it improper for a lady to appear at a theatre or any smart gathering without being correctly gowned and smartly coiffed. Since the commencement of hostilities, on the contrary, it has been held to be incorrect to attend a public function in other than a simple garb. One hears murmurs and even open criticism now of anyone who is at all elegantly attired.

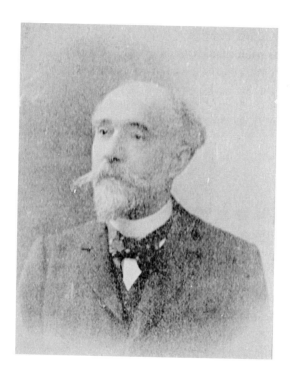

Figure 24. A Portrait of Marcel Grateau, Inventor of 'Marcel' Waving. From Long, *Traité complet et illustré de l'ondulation.*

This is all due to the spirited discussions which have been going on in the Press regarding the question of whether luxury is necessary or unnecessary at this moment. There has been no decision arrived at, and the partisans both for and against remain, as formerly, divided into two groups of about equal force.

Every time a fashionable lady employs workpeople who are engaged in trades *de luxe*, even if it be with the laudable intention of coming to their aid, those on the one side cry 'Shame.' In the same way, whenever through lack of clients the members of the trades *de luxe* find themselves compelled to close their establishments, and in consequence to discharge a crowd of employees of both sexes, those on the other side in their turn, cry 'Disastrous.'

I, myself, am on the side of the latter, as, in my opinion, it is they who are right. No matter how grave the situation may be, one ought never to prevent persons who have the money from spending it, and even generously. And as employees in general, and particularly those in the higher class businesses, are above accepting charity, it is only fair to allow them to exchange the product of their efforts for the money offered by those who have been more privileged by fortune.

In any case, who can say where simplicity finishes and luxury begins? Must it be that in order to avoid hurting the feelings of extreme puritans, the affluent members of the community, who have always been elegant in their appearance, must transform themselves into apparent beggars?

The co-ordination of styles in toilettes can no more be accomplished than the elimination of class distinction. One finds nothing absolutely the same in the world. In Nature as amongst human beings nothing is exactly similar. Even human hair itself always shows some slight difference. Therefore, how can it be said that all coiffures must be alike. There are ladies of taste who, when simply gowned, have the air of little queens, on account of natural or acquired personal charm. Must we forbid other persons, not perhaps naturally gifted, to study their appearance, and attempt to secure equal or some part of that charm? Must it be counted a crime to appear decently dressed, especially amongst those who have the money, and who on all sides are being solicited for orders?

No, women (even the most coquettish) do not overlook that we are at war, and there is no need of reminding them of the fact. Since the gravity of the situation demands it, they have themselves renounced all the extravagant exaggerations of pre-war days – unfortunately for us. A large number of workpeople are already unemployed through this self-denial, and others have heavy liabilities to shoulder.

Therefore, let us continue to learn and perfect ourselves in the various branches of our profession, which will continue to exist in spite of all influences of war. We have the duty of transmitting intact to those who come after us the professional heritage that was bequeathed to us by our predecessors, and if possible we must make it prosperous. It is on account of this sacred duty that the Parisian coiffeurs are at this moment straining every effort to keep the Hairdressing Academies open, notwithstanding all the difficulties that are met with, and they are trying to stimulate study and efficiency in our art by encouraging pupils regularly to attend the various schools. Though the feminine element predominates at the schools for the moment, and the principal study is Marcel waving, one, nevertheless, can see in the academies interesting designs in coiffures, which fact augurs well for the future of our Trade.

March 1917: Professional Possibilities for Ladies Hairdressers

Our trade shows marked progress, in spite of the enormous difficulties that have had to be overcome since the commencement of the war. If we examine separately the three or four specialities which are of interest to most coiffeurs de dames, we shall be able to realise the changes that have taken place since then.

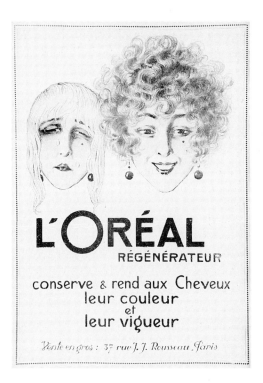

Figure 25. 'L'Oréal Régénérateur – to give your hair colour and body', an advertisement for L'Oréal hair colouring. From *La Coiffure de Paris*, 1922.

Hair Dyes

For instance, hair dyes were, to a certain extent, neglected formerly, but more recently numerous persons have taken up this branch of the trade seriously – and prospered thereby. Illustrated manuals, well compiled and produced, and very comprehensive, have been published for hairdressers' use, containing the best recipes and methods of application. At the same time, our own trade journals have contained long articles on the subject, explaining how necessary it is for hairdressers to take up this lucrative branch of the trade, and enumerating the benefits it is possible to obtain from it.

Clients have been attracted by the various prominent advertisements, and have at once placed their confidence in henna, persuaded that the application of the extract of this plant will be followed by good results. The liquid dyes are sold for all purposes – for the beard, for gentlemen's hair, and for those little services that clients who are travelling, or who reside at some distance from their hairdressers, must see to for themselves. But practically all the preparations that are made at the trade saloons contain more or less henna; at all events, they always pass for henna, without distinction, as they are all mixed with boiling water, and are applied to the head hot. Why not, then, let us proclaim unceasingly that henna is a marvelous plant, tinting rapidly, without any danger, and giving any desired shade.

Hair Waving

After a thirty years' continuous vogue, which is really a record in the history of fashion, it makes us wonder how our ancestors managed without waving their hair. No doubt there has been an evolution in waving, but in whatever method the hair is dressed, it still takes the form of waves, and it is this method that produces for us the best returns, and in their turn, clients profit by the elegant effects obtained.

Marcel's great invention has been democratised and popularised in each of its branches by all classes, and to-day has penetrated everywhere.

Now there is not even a modest work-girl or shop-assistant who does not resort to its infinite possibilities, and the lady of fashion is hard put to it to render her appearance distinct from, and superior to, the appearance of her more humble sister. She may change the aspect of the waves, but she cannot resign herself to abandoning them altogether.

The most exclusive waves are now excessively wide, supple and brilliant. The greatest durability is obtained by the application of heat, principally by means of an electric apparatus, which bids fair to having a brilliant future before it. Another method of obtaining those luxurious coiffures which are half curls and half waves, consists in waving their hair with curl papers; and those who are able and willing to pay for this method are themselves repaid by the excellent results obtained. It is all merely a question of time and money.

May 1917: Is Ladies' Hair to be Shortened?

Attracted by several styles of hairdressing, which seem to have been on the increase since the war, the smart set are again talking of cutting their hair. Some have already done so; others are following their example daily.

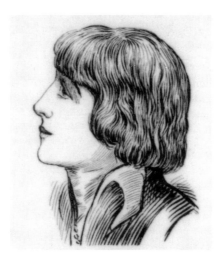

Figure 26. The 'mode à la Jeanne d'Arc', a sketch of the coiffure of actress Eve Lavallière, who first made it famous in 1909. From *HWJS*, May 1917.

It is notable that this style of hairdressing comes into vogue periodically, but rarely does it become general. Perhaps on this occasion it will be otherwise, now that it is not a question of cutting the hair short like a man's (a horrible fashion which 'masculine women' have at different times adopted), but of leaving it about a foot in length, so that it can be elegantly dressed according to the present day modes.

A good hairdresser can obtain very smart effects from hair about a foot in length, and in any case Parisiennes who have their hair waved twice weekly will most likely not have much to cut, if this fashion becomes general. I do not blame anyone, but simply mention what everyone can see for themselves: that ladies' hair is visibly becoming shorter. Posticheurs are taking this matter up seriously. They are commencing to exhibit in their windows and to illustrate in their catalogues such models, the extremities of which fall in ringlets, as well as the hair on the crown and temples. A dozen or so actresses (principally those of the music hall stage, such as Polaire, Mistinguette, Colette, Willy, etc.) who up to the present have worn their hair in ringlets are now dressing it on the crown.

When the hair is freshly curled it has [a nice] appearance, but a few days later the hair stands out like the quills of a hedgehog, and the more frizzed and woolly it is, the more it amuses the public. It would seem that the success of wearers of this style develops as their hair becomes more untidy.

Some, however, take more pains, and when their hair commences to get untidy they dress it so carefully that one cannot perceive that it is not of ordinary length. It is this style that has commenced the vogue of cutting the hair, and after all, why hesitate to shorten the hair if it can still be dressed in many modes.

There is a good majority of people who take no notice of styles or coiffures or fashions. For example, take Eve Lavallière, who has for probably 30 years played in the most important French theatres (from this it may be conjectured that she is no longer young). However, thanks to the effects of henna, she is now playing the part of a young girl of 15, her hair cut to the neck, as she always wears it in ordinary life as at the theatre. This is called the Joan of Arc style of coiffure – that is to say, the style that ladies often select for their children's hair.

It may be remarked that modern women are not all stupid enough to adopt such a style. True, but since Fashion has decreed such short skirts, we must ask ourselves where feminine eccentricities will cease.

The Joan of Arc coiffure reminds me that, according to history, actresses were not the only people who wore their hair short. Ninon d'Enclos (one of the most celebrated beauties of the 17th century) wore her hair in short graceful curls all her life. She died at the age of 85, still very beautiful.

Marie Antoinette, Queen of France, also had her hair cut short as a child, and always wore curls. She also was beautiful and a coquette. It was to her that our first ladies' hairdressers owed their reputation, as previously it was women who dressed ladies' hair. It is perhaps unnecessary to recall that this was the period when hairdressers commenced to make use of curling irons. A little later, Mme. Récamier, and all the ladies of Napoleon's Court, wore their hair in short curls.

June 1917: Ladies' Hairdressing Seen in the Parisian Academies

When one examines closely the general evolution which is going on, a tendency towards a simpler and more democratic mode of living can be discerned. In bygone days there were both the academic language and the language of the multitude, which was much more rudimentary. Now-a-days we speak so much that there is not time to cultivate a polished style, to study one's phrases and weigh one's words. Besides, academicians are scarce, and ordinary writers very numerous. It is the same with clothes. When, some thirty years ago, I was an employee of a high-class hairdresser, my fellow workers and I were not permitted to interview lady clients except we were garbed in a frock coat, white tie and silk hat. At the present day, so long as one is clean, one can go anywhere in a lounge suit and fancy tie. It is of no importance now whether one wears a beard or is clean shaven, whereas formerly nobody could realise the confidence which a big black beard inspired, when one had to attend in a professional capacity.

Then there were very complicated, voluminous, and much ornamented coiffures, which were reserved for prize competitions and fashion plates; there were also the simple and practical coiffures which were dressed on the clients' own heads. Now everything is changed. The instructors at the academies have retired one after the other, and with them have taken the secret of the multiple interlacings, the intricate manipulations of knots, curls, and torsades that have become almost useless since the invention of Marcel waving, which in itself is such an ornamentation to the hair. There is hardly any difference in the coiffure of to-day as seen in the fashion journals, and the everyday styles as worn by ladies. The only distinction consists in a variation according to the part of a city in which a particular business may be situated and the social status of the clients themselves.

If we study the styles of the various young professors in the different technical schools, we can discern at once the class of clients on whom they attend.

[The less expensive coiffures] have no added postiche and occupy from 30 to 45 minutes to dress. They have been executed by young professors who are employed in different houses where there is much hairdressing done at a cost of about two francs, waving included.

July 1917: The Female Ladies' Hairdressers of Paris

It is well known that in pre-war days there were not more than ten lady hairdressers in Paris. At present there are over 2,000, and careful inquiry amongst private schools and masters brings to light the following statistics:—

During the thirty months of war there have been trained and certified, on an average, seventy pupils per month. This makes 2,100, without taking into consideration those who have taught themselves, and who are therefore

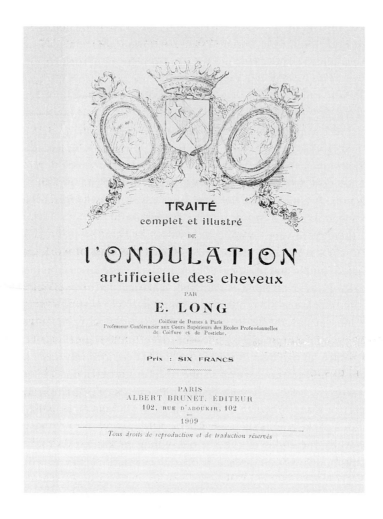

Figure 27. Frontispiece of Emile Long's *Traité complet et illustré de l'ondulation*.

not enrolled. Each one of these students pays on an average £10 and works about two months in order to learn waving and obtain her diploma. The age of these pupils usually varies between 13 and 40 years. It is estimated that at least half of this continent are young ladies between the ages of 13 and 20 (hairdressers' daughters and otherwise), and the other half consist of the wives of hairdressers who have been killed or mobilised or are missing, and also a minority who were not connected with our Trade formerly.

It is very interesting to watch these young girls at work – in their eagerness to learn. The ambition to get on (which is such a powerful asset) assists them more than the tuition of their teachers. The long, numerous, and practical sessions do the rest. The very young learn very quickly. They are not distracted by other people's conversations, and moreover they are more closely watched. Some ten years ago I published as a curiosity in the *Traité d'Ondulation* a photograph of a young girl of 13 who had obtained at this early age her diploma in waving, and was shown working on a small stool. I called her 'the small prodigy,' because she was the only girl of that age who could wave a client's hair nicely and quickly. But nowadays prodigies are numerous; I know more than fifty. There are many girls, with their hair still in plaits and not yet 15, who earn from 6 to 8 francs per day, and who, in order to gain this sum, must wave the hair of 10 to 15 clients daily. Wavers who are a little older obtain about double, and to do this they must wave at least 25 heads of hair in a day. It will be seen by this that it is a golden age for wavers, but it will also be understood that this class of work cannot be continued for long, as it is very tiring.

The average charge for having one's hair waved by a lady waver is 1 franc. It must be understood that this price does not include any waving at the back of the head, and in the front and at the sides only one thickness of hair. The time occupied is usually from 15 to 20 minutes. Through continual practice the girls finally are able to master the most rebellious hair, and they are proud to show the corns and blisters that they have on the hands. One often seen them quite tired out; with a bandage round their aching wrists. But what of that? The work is lucrative, and experience is being gained. Later on they will act as others have done formerly, so as to avoid so much hard work (and possibly the hospital); they will increase their charges in proportion to their capabilities.

There is a great improvement in the work done now to what was seen at the commencement of the war, when the thousands of employees who were called up had to be immediately replaced. The models vary very little; all the customers have to be satisfied with practically the same style of coiffure. The models do not change very much either in the different firms. This is on account of all the wavers having been taught at the same schools – as there are very few of them. However, they do not hesitate, and do their work very rapidly. The girls who have been taught by coiffeurs make much softer and larger waves than the others, and are so adept at arranging the hair and executing those little etceteras which go towards making a smart coiffure that they seem to have a promising future before them. Finally, they have great confidence in themselves, and are proud of their work. One of them recommends her clients to take her walks bare-headed, with only a sunshade, remarking that this is good for the hair, when in reality the object in view is to create admiration for the waving.

August 1917: Postiche *de Luxe*

The general outline of the present-day coiffure (the fashion is practically the same at this moment in all cases) is very high on the summit of the head, and flat all round, with very large, soft waves. This style of headdress is becoming very general; present appearances indicate that it has come to stay for a long period; and certainly it gives satisfaction to most ladies. Hairdressers realise this, and improve on their work more and more, the styles being both becoming and practical. In the domain of fashion, as in politics, the minority always ends by siding with the majority.

It must be understood that all classes of hair will not lend themselves to these styles of hairdressing. Some hair may be too long, other hair too short; some of it grows too low, other hair too high; and other hair, again, refuses to turn in the right direction. For this reason there has been patented a new invention called the 'postiche envellopeur.' This no more resembles the former postiche than the moon resembles the sun, but here we see the superiority of specialities in this as in every other branch of human activity. Already many hairdressers have been compelled to neglect their usual styles of postiche in order to devote more time to the 'postiche envellopeur,' much in the same way as physicians one by one give their attention to one subject as a special study, instead of going in for medicine in general. And the result is as may be expected. In the hands of modern artists the manufacture of 'postiche envellopeurs' has already acquired such a high degree of perfection that it would be difficult to improve on it.

All hairdressers are not in a position to take up this style of postiche, neither are the charges within the scope of everyone, as they commence at 400 francs for ordinary shades.

September 1917: Something New for the Coming Season

Now that the holiday season has arrived, the greater number of the *maisons de coiffure pour dames* in Paris are closed. Even in those which remain open for business the bulk of the work that has to be done is delegated to just a few female members of the staff. Shop windows are empty, or nearly so, and the wax figures enveloped in paper; the principals of the establishments are in the Army or on holiday; only a very few houses, indeed, show anything approaching their customary activity.

Since the war this short hair, waved or slightly frizzed, has increased very much. The face, and even the entire head, are now garnished by the short locks.

October 1917: Postiche Produced in Paris by the Large Wholesale Postiche Houses

Associated with the hair merchants in two powerful associations, the wholesale postiche manufacturers have jointly decided to raise their prices so as to unify their tariffs for materials, work, redressing, etc. Now that so many coiffeurs and posticheurs have been called to the Army and been compelled, consequently, to leave their establishments in the charge, in many instances, of inexperienced women, the wholesale manufacturers of postiche have received a tremendous amount of extra work. This will be easily understood, considering the large number of hairdressers' wives who, not being themselves posticheuses, have been compelled to send all postiche belonging to their clients which need remodelling or repairing to the wholesale postiche supply houses.

There are those wholesale manufacturers of postiche who employ the best materials and turn out beautifully made postiche for hairdressers, and there are others, who were formerly employed in large warehouses, haberdashery establishments, etc., who have started as postiche manufacturers in the same way as they would have commenced in any line of business, with the sole end in view of increasing their capital – in other words, to make money.

Those who manufacture postiche at cheap rates and in considerable quantities do so for large and small fancy dealers, retail perfumers, haberdashery establishments, etc., in fact, every one of the tradespeople who are competitors of the hairdresser; and, ultimately, it is they who by their inartistic, inelegant and defective productions create amongst the public a disgust for postiche work generally.

In order to enable them to produce cheaply, these manufacturers naturally employ common hair, made up by apprentices in the charge of forewomen, who have been specially trained for this class of work The curled hair used being very unstable, the postiche is dressed dry, when the undulations obtained are strongly held up with cord, damped with a vaporiser and then placed in a very hot oven.

There are others who simply employ glue diluted in boiling water for their postiche work. The effect of this is good, and permits of the postiche being displayed in windows or stored in boxes for long periods without one hair getting disarranged. Such postiches can be dusted with a feather-duster without their effect being damaged in the least.

Yes, but once this effect has gone, the postiche has a poor appearance, just the same as, say, cheap calico containing a great deal of dressing, after it has been washed.

November 1917: The Latest Headdresses for the New Millinery

If the hairdressing executed at the opening demonstrations of the principal hairdressing schools of Paris may be accepted as embodying what is most up to-date in fashion, it can safely be asserted that the high headdress maintains its position as the prevailing mode. In fact, not only was the coiffure dressed above the crown to be seen more or less generally – it was exhibited practically to the exclusion of all other styles of hairdressing.

The ornamentation in nearly all instances consisted of combs, pins and barrettes *made of wood*, which are the latest novelty. For several months the comb manufacturers have realised that the supplies of the ordinary raw material necessary for their products was rapidly becoming exhausted. So they followed the course of substituting wood which is naturally hard, or artificially hardened, and when manufactured from this, hair ornaments are light and can be perfectly decorated.

This year the coiffeurs have invited the leading modistes to take part in the hairdressing classes. Has this been done by way of gallantry? Or is it not rather in order to inaugurate a desirable understanding between the two industries? Whatever the reason, the modistes have responded and in addition to attending have had many complimentary things to say to the hairdressers in reference to their professional efforts.

During the first six months of 1917, the Parisian women honoured the arrival in France of the first contingent of the American Army by adopting hats which were exactly similar, in style and colour, to those worn by their brave Allies from across the Atlantic. The peaked cap, and the large flat brim, which affords protection from the sun – not too much in evidence this summer, however – give to the wearer a pleasing appearance. Unfortunately, these rigid hats, like all of a similar character, were sold by the hatters, and the modistes were considerably upset, because they considered that the hatters made sufficient money out of their sales to gentlemen. Women's hats, they maintain, should not be rigid and should be sold by the modistes. That is why the latter have this Autumn been anxious to be first in introducing the new styles.

To the somewhat surprised – and perhaps also somewhat deceived – coiffeurs, the modistes, with their usual seductive smile, have explained that these styles will be advantageous to every one. For instance, they are high and soft, and permit of being made still higher if need be. Then the hats extend low over the forehead and thus, it is urged, fulfil a desirable purpose, for in order to discern the effect produced by her remarks the lady is compelled to raise her head to look in her companion's eyes, much as if she were endeavouring to track an aeroplane in the sky. I inquired of one of these modistes if she would be good enough to remover her hat, in order that I could see the kind of 'skilfully executed coiffure' that the hat 'protected' in her case. This she did readily – although these large hats are rather heavy – previously explaining, however, that her own coiffure was not very elaborate. 'Besides,' she added, 'modistes generally dress their hair quite plainly.' But now that the modistes have attended our professional schools and have witnessed the hairdressing which is taught and executed there, they will no doubt convey a better impression of it to their clients, who are also ours.

December 1917: New Style of Postiche by Leading Paris Specialists

It has been apparent for some time that the leading posticheurs of Paris have been meeting with considerable commercial success – due more and more to a complete alteration in the style of their specialities. We do not now see anything else but these large postiches in the shop windows of the modern and leading specialists. On the other hand, the large *magasins de nouveautés* which now have hairdressing saloons for ladies, the manicure establishments, all the perfumers and the bulk of the ordinary hairdressers, exhibit a quantity of small pieces of postiche too frizzy and waved to please the elegant Paris-iennes. Nevertheless there is a demand for such work, as there are many coquettes possessing no personal taste and to whom it would be impossible to sell postiche of the latest design and make.

9

January 1918: Fashion in the Hairdressing Schools for the Wounded Victims of the War

Since it is usual at the commencement of the year to express one's good wishes, let us in the first place have a kind thought for those who have nobly borne their part militarily in the defence of their country, whilst we professionally have safeguarded the interests of the Trade to which we mutually belong. Let us take steps to ensure that when our *confrères* return after the cessation of hostilities, they will not have to bear fresh hardships where it is possible for them to resume their ordinary work or their customary business affairs. Our efforts, collective and individual, can greatly assist in the accomplishment of this purpose; let us therefore at once make all the efforts to this end that are within our power, each within our particular sphere. The economists teach us that it is not alone by personal carefulness and self-denial that we shall help to restore prosperity after the war, but chiefly by work and by production.

Independent of the Trade schools and associations, and of the private academies, there have already been formed in Paris two schools which are reserved for the wounded and for the widows of the war. A third is in process of formation, and more are likely to follow. Some hundreds of maimed soldiers, formerly belonging to every imaginable vocation, have been able to learn in these special schools to shave, cut hair, wave, dress ladies' hair, dye, make postiche, and do other hair work, each according to his particular infirmity and ability. A number are already established on their own account, whilst others have been engaged as employees by various houses. All are gaining a livelihood in their new calling. Others, again, are continuing to perfect themselves in the various branches of the profession. Nothing is wanting in these schools in material, appliances, teachers or benevolent patrons. In fact, everything and everybody necessary have been at the disposal of the students from morning till night and every day during the past two years.

[Among these pupils I saw] two different classes of hairdressing – the 'coiffeur' style and the 'public' style. The first is generally that of the new hairdressers who practised as barbers before the war, and who have been imbued with the Trade spirit for a long time. The second style is the sort of hairdressing which clients dress themselves. The latter type of coiffures are executed by the students who were not in our profession before the war and to whom the classical methods of our Trade academies are unknown.

The latter style is certainly more artistic and more natural; it is always preferred by those of our clients who wish to be *bien coiffées*. The first may impart a more delicate effect to the elegant ladies who prefer waving to hairdressing – those who wish to show that they have incurred the expense of a visit to their hairdresser – by the large number of waves that their hair bears. But ladies of this category usually frequent the cheap hairdressing establishments, in which undulation is the one consideration, and to which all the efforts of the staff are devoted, where prominent waves are the one thing to which importance is attached and which are the pride and the hall-mark of the house.

This may be all right, but it is not always sufficient. The specialist in waving can live; the true coiffeur can make provision for his later years, because he has several strings to his bow. By intelligent handling he develops his trade into a lucrative commercial concern with more than one department and possibility of success when necessity arises. Then, too, the exercise of his profession is infinitely more varied and interesting. Let us not decry or detract from the merits of waving, because it is that which brings clients to us, but at the same time do not let us remain content with waving solely.

February 1918: The Two Styles of Hairdressing

Dealing with the subject of the results produced by the teaching in the hairdressing schools of Paris, I explained and illustrated last month the general tendency of hairdressing styles amongst the two categories of pupils – those who already know a little about it and those who were complete strangers to our profession. I am obliged to return to this somewhat important topic as the same distinctive tendencies towards the 'hairdresser' style in the one case and the 'public' style in the other are clearly discernible also amongst the master hairdressers of our Capital.

Never, perhaps, has the 'public' style, which is naturally the more modern, vied so powerfully with the classical or 'hairdresser' style, which is the one followed by the older hairdressing firms and by the generality of hairdressers who frequent (or have frequented) the Trade schools. All ladies who have the least independence of mind dislike our professional system, and even show resentment against our profession. Nevertheless, they continue to

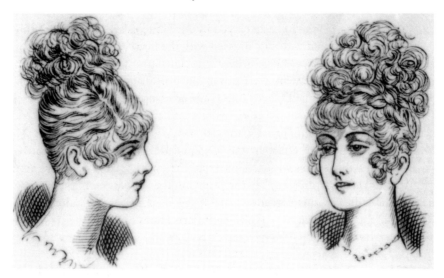

Figure 28. Two examples of the so-called 'Public Styles' by the 'modernist' coiffeur, M. François. From *HWJS*, February 1918.

patronise our shops, but on one condition – viz., that we provide in place of the hackneyed academic style of hairdressing modes which embrace some novelty and originality.

It cannot be wondered at, therefore, that the tendency of the modern client of wealth and social position is to transfer her patronage to those hairdressing firms which are up-to-date in their methods and which dress the hair on the lines which conform to present-day tastes. These houses naturally are not very numerous yet; we in Paris do not number even half a dozen amongst the two thousand who cater for ladies' hairdressing, but the success which has already made itself apparent is sufficient to encourage others to follow the example set by the few.

The admitted head of this new school of Paris coiffeurs is M. François, to whom I have often referred in the *Supplement*, and whose personality will not be lost sight of, as he is the instigator of a trade revolution which has started since the outbreak of the war, and which promises to be fruitful in its effects and influence. M. François works single-handed in quite a small shop. But his charges are very high – the highest, in fact, in Paris – and as his *clientèle* increases so his charges rise. Before his narrow shop window, which cannot hold more than three figures and generally has two, you can see every day as many hairdressers as clients. The former are attracted by curiosity – by what has become almost the magic of the name 'François' – just as years ago Marcel's show window in the Rue de l'Echelle was the magnet which drew members of the craft from all parts of the city and even of France. The two or three figures which are displayed by M. François are always tastefully and well dressed – that is to say, dressed with the large postiche which is his speciality, very *à la mode*, and fresh in conception and treatment. These figures, in fact, are always so *chic* and enticing that passers-by purchase postiche without even trying it – simply on the general effect of the figure in the window.

When the war is ended I propose to travel to London and bring M. François with me (as I did M. Marcel years ago), so that he can give a demonstration of his hairdressing. The extraordinary taste of this man, who was originally an artiste musician and took up our profession quite accidentally when he was thirty years of age, will, I am sure, be appreciated by our British colleagues just as much as it has been by the elegant Parisiennes.

March 1918: The Three Principal Coiffures for 1918

What is the fashion in hairdressing? Decidedly it is the high style of coiffure – that can be stated confidently in a few words. But there are several ways of interpreting what is meant by that phrase. It would be impossible to enumerate all the different forms of coiffures dressed high on the head that one sees at the present day, nearly all of which are *à la mode*, and yet do not resemble each other very closely.

It is necessary first to take into account the different grades of society. For instance, the older ladies of social position dress their hair quite simply, whilst the more youthful section are more anxious after effect – a grand effect – without being too scrupulous in the matter of taste. Amongst the humbler classes we find the classical and relatively modest style of coiffure, with waves and rolled chignon or knot chignon. In the domain of the music-halls and theatre-concerts, where are to be found more eccentric and extravagant proclivities, we see headdresses in which the hair is cut short and curled in quite a disorderly style, being sometimes left entirely free and sometimes bound together with a ribbon or a turban of soft material, and sometimes separated into tufts or clusters and arranged in the most comical ways.

April 1918: Paris Fashion in Ladies' Hairdressing

Our English and American colleagues frequently honour us with very flattering remarks, amongst which we often notice the following phrase: 'Paris is leading; we are following.'

If this is really the case, it seems rather strange that at least a few of the hairdressers in the Allied countries have not followed the general movement in favour of the high coiffure, with very little fulness at the sides and at the nape of the neck.

It is remarkable that elegant Parisiennes will not have their hair waved in any other than large, soft undulations, though a certain number of hairdressers try to impress on clients of the Allied countries that, on the contrary, it is very narrow, severe waves that are the most modern.

As will be readily understood, all this concerns the most elegant clientèle. With the lower grade of customer frequenting the cheaper class of establishment, one sees curls that are too frizzy and waves which are much too pronounced. Certainly as regards elegance the high mode of coiffure takes first place.

May 1918: Shortening the Hair

In Paris there are specialist wavers who are hostile to postiche, and posticheurs who do not encourage the use of waving. The consequence is that clients have to decide for themselves which system of hairdressing they will adopt; that is to say, whether they will accord their patronage to the waver who is always disposed to cut the hair in order to assure more waving with the iron, or to the posticheur who never cuts his clients' hair, but covers it with curled postiche. In both cases the lady who desires that her coiffure shall be fashionable is obliged to spend money – daily, or at any rate frequently, in small amounts if she has her own hair waved, or in one relatively high sum if she has one postiche or several. I say 'several postiches' designedly, as it is not by any means rare to see ladies of elegance who adopt several styles of coiffure and even several shades of hair – for their own apartment in the morning, for outdoor wear in the afternoon, and for the various forms of artificial light in the evening.

In all cases coiffures of short hair (or in imitation of short hair) are the rage at the present moment. And in the case of this style of hairdressing, as in all others, it is the ladies whom this fashion suits well who force it into prominence and make it popular; they exert a power of propaganda with which reams of paper and hours of argument bear no effective comparison. On the other hand, inordinate exaggeration by persons to whom the style is totally unsuited exert an opposite influence by generating dislike and disgust.

One must always bear in mind that in order to attract a clientèle, each lady's particular tastes, the exigencies of the fashion, the individual type of face, the thickness of the hair, and even the state of the temperature have all to be carefully considered. In the warm weather everything that is light and soft is naturally preferred to what is heavy and cumbersome, or what appears to be. With voile gowns and the tulle or light straw millinery that the smart set wear now, which is, or appears to be, as fleecy and intangible as a cloud, it is necessary that the coiffure should harmonise; and in order to obtain this soft effect certain ladies employ means which are at once the simplest and most radical – that is, to have their own hair cut and waved so as to assume a really light effect. The other method, which gives a light appearance and is very popular, as it allows ladies to retain their own hair intact, is to cover the head with a sort of bonnet of waved postiche that can be taken off at will. This course is perhaps the most prudent, as styles change very rapidly.

June 1918: Ladies' Hairdressing as seen at Leading Parisian Dressmakers

Being a ladies' hairdresser, I am a member of a Committee which was formed just before the war with the intention (or, to be more exact, the pretension) of directing the fashion in ladies' hairdressing. As a journalist I have no faith

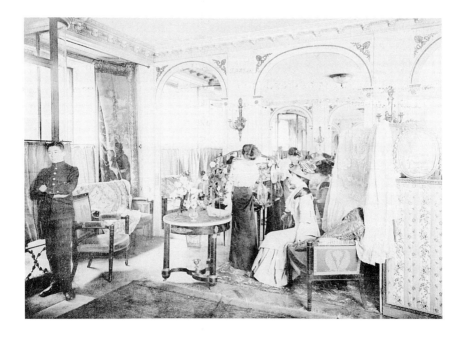

Figure 29. A peek inside the exclusive salon of the *Maison Paquin*. From *Les créateurs de la mode.*

in the possibilities of this Committee, which is still in existence and is composed of eminent modistes, milliners, hairdressers, etc. I have no faith in it because I realise that Fashion will not allow herself to be influenced and directed as easily as some would have us believe, and more especially by a mere Committee.

However, as this Committee does exist it must do something to justify its existence, so meetings are held occasionally, ideas are exchanged, different points of view are examined, and a number of models are designed for submission to our respective professions. After these meetings we disperse to our individual businesses, and once there no further heed or thought is given to the decisions which have been arrived at; the usual course is to forget them almost at once when one is confronted with the necessities of practical everyday business affairs.

The visits that I have paid to several of the leading dressmakers have shown that not one of them has followed the decision of the Committee [as regards their coiffures]. The young girls who are employed to display the new creations of these artist dressmakers are not allowed to dress their hair as they wish during the hours when (like actresses playing their parts) they fulfil their duties. There is a small dressing-room reserved for them, where they complete their toilet after the directions of the firm by whom they are employed, so as to show off, with the maximum amount of *éclat* and effect, the costumes that are offered for sale. It is not their fault, therefore, but the fault of the proprietor, if they do not dress their hair in the style agreed on by the committee, or if the selected headdress is replaced by one which is directly opposite in style.

July 1918: Parisian Milliners' Hairdressing Styles

It has occurred to me that this month it will not be inappropriate if I deal with the head-dresses that are representative of the modes to be met with in the principal millinery establishments, which we are bound to take into account.

As a matter of fact, as the annals of feminine coquetry record, their profession and ours mainly proceed side by side – sometimes together in harmonious inter-working, at other times separately in competition and rivalry.

In this way the famous coiffeur Léonard worked for a long period with the great modiste Rose Bertin in the adornment of the person of Marie Antoinette. Léonard accumulated a large fortune, which in the end he lost in an unfortunate theatrical enterprise; Mlle. Bertin terminated her commercial venture in modes by going into bankruptcy with a deficit of two million francs, which was an extraordinary amount at that epoch, and at least worthy of note even in these days.

Until towards the year 1890 the coiffeur occupied a position of superiority compared with that of the modiste. But, of course, ladies' hairdressers were then much less numerous than they are to-day. Coiffeurs first disposed of their creations in postiche, etc., to the clients, who afterwards consulted their milliners as to what to wear with them. Now it is the reverse. Milliners may not be more numerous than hairdressers, but there are among them some real artists who are determined to outdo us by the variety of the seductive models that they are continually creating. These are immediately copied by their competitors and sold at cheap prices by the large stores. Of course they have every opportunity of making their models successful, as they have at their command all kinds of flowers, feathers, stones, ribbons and other material, straw, lace, etc. They can employ all these in the most diverse colours and obtain the most charming effects.

Designers frequent the principal museums and libraries in order to collect material and illustrations from the records of former fashions. They then produce sketches of hats suitable for modern wear founded on the outstanding and most attractive features of the ancient headgear. Afterwards, with these designs before them, selected and perhaps improved by the *grande modiste*, the *premières* of the establishments apply their imaginative faculties to the task of producing a number of different models. Then follows a fresh selection and many modifications, following which the *grande modiste* submits several of the models to her best clients, and on their criticism and suggestion finally founds the definite styles.

But though interesting and useful, all this is apart from the actual object of this article, viz., to show how the leading milliners regard ladies' hair-dressing. Generally speaking, they dress the hair very simply and solidly, which is quite natural when it is remembered that they try on some twenty or thirty hats a day.

August 1918: French Army Women's Hairdressing

Little that is new in ladies' hairdressing is to be seen in Paris during the quiet summer months. Therefore it may be well if I make this an opportunity of showing in the present article the more characteristic of head-dresses which are being worn by the many Frenchwomen who are engaged on work con-nected with the military, the infirmaries, automobiles, etc.

There is nothing official about the present types of ladies' hairdressing.

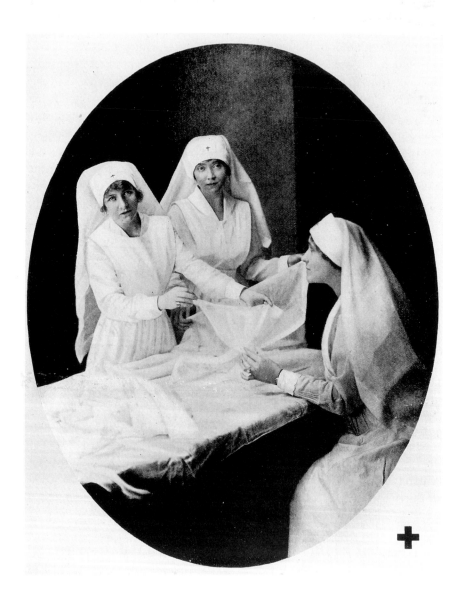

Figure 30.

The military regulations which stipulate for a definite style of men's hair-cutting, have not yet been extended so as to provide for one certain way of wearing the hair by women. Each section of the service has its own particular style, by which it is distinguished from the others. The 'bonnet japonnais' (Japanese cap) appears to me to be the one which is the most general.

Influenced, no doubt, by the present vogue in hairdressing, and also by what is clearly most convenient and comfortable during the hot weather, a large number of the women who are engaged on war service in the open air have shortened their tresses. Others whose time is spent in doing sedentary work have not shown the same preference for short hair, probably because they cannot be continually going to the expert waver; so their efforts have been devoted to devising a coiffure which is practical and serviceable for their purpose – that is to say, one that is neat and firm, which they can dress themselves, and which can be worn under the cap or other headgear.

Often we see with what relief and pleasure the military women alter [their coiffures] when doffing their uniforms during brief periods of respite from service. Usually their first call is at the hairdresser's, where before the mirrors, and with the aid of the complicated arsenal of aesthetic contrivances provided in our salons, they soon revive their taste for coquetry and also their appearance of the time when elegance was their sole preoccupation. Naturally we readily make them conversant with the changes that have taken place in the dressing of the hair, show them the latest productions in combs and postiche, and demonstrate anything that is new in the treatment and embellishment of the face. There have been introduced creams and powders which are lightly tinted; the rouges are of brick-colour foundation; and even the blondes now use these special preparations, which give a tanned or sunburnt appearance.

September 1918: Present-day Parisian Coiffures

If we are under the necessity of taking an active part in our saloon or business attendance – that is to say, to work a great deal with our hands – all our attention is absorbed by this manual labour, and it is impossible for us to apply our efforts and our initiative to more profitable tasks. In this case, we secure more or less what is necessary for our existence, but little beyond. On the other hand, when we are not compelled to apply ourselves to purely manual labour we can devote our mental faculties to the improvement of our productions, to the organisation and the advancement of our businesses; we can closely examine the hair of our clients and suggest either suitable and needed treatment or articles which they require for their improvement. In this case we derive much more pecuniary benefit, with less work.

The timid ones, [whose method] consists of working with their hands, personally and solely, commit a grave error, because they lose both time and money, two things which can never be recovered. Moreover, they may easily find themselves ruined one day, for they are at the mercy of the slightest illness or accident. In any case their period of apparent success cannot endure for very long, for conditions and circumstances change frequently and strength and energy are rapidly used up.

Another great advantage for a ladies' hairdresser in not being too closely confined to manual labour is that he is able to keep close observation on what is occurring from time to time in fashions generally, and also to inform himself promptly as to what is new in the world of fashion and society. All of such information is, of course, precious; it incites emulation, courage and ideas which are always profitable. It is an admirable method, because of the impulse and information obtainable from it, to follow the exhibitions of the *grandes elegantes* and the productions of the coiffeurs of renown. There is no better way of keeping oneself abreast of the incessant evolution of Fashion, and of being able to apply to one's own business the most characteristic tendencies of the times. I have adopted this course; I often exhaust myself in the school rooms of the different Parisian societies.

October 1918: Curls Returning to Fashion

The little wisp of hair, which in contour reminded one of the comma, or the snail, that before the war ladies delighted to see hanging in front of the ear, has since gradually grown in proportions. For is not Fashion often fed on exaggeration and eccentricity? And then there was the problem how the lady of elegance and position was to be distinctive and different in her appearance from her humble sister, under the hats which were thrust down over the head. There was but one way – to resort to the wearing of little curls. And this is the style at present.

All modern posticheurs are very ingenious and comprise many real artistes, whose capabilities enable them to produce models more beautiful even than natural ones, or at all events as beautiful as the most attractive to be seen anywhere and very rare reproductions of Nature. Their work at times creates quite a sensation, and therefore it is not surprising that clients are captivated by their models and consent to pay fantastic prices for them. But what effort, time and highly-paid employees are required for the production of these little capillary marvels! I know of clever female workers who are paid twenty francs per day and who take eight days to make a postiche of hair which is very rare, and in consequence very costly. Afterwards the principal of the establishment must again take the postiche in hand, dress it and add the *chic* finish and embellishment which constitute its characteristic quality. Then it must be tried on the client, modified if and where necessary, and made complete for its final acceptance. What is the value of such a production? Really it has no fixed price.

Those of us who sell postiche by weight or measurement cannot form an idea of the difficulties, care and artistic effort which are required for *postiche d'art*. The ordinary commercial houses sell cheaper in order to sell more. They form the greater number, and they copy in their way the ideas and models of the leading professional artistes.

November 1918: Up-to-date Coiffures and Postiche in Paris

Parisian work-girls and female employees generally have now all acquired the habit of attending the hairdresser's, and nearly all for waving. The cheap *salons d'ondulation* have large and increasing connections and are open until as late as nine o'clock at night in the populous quarters. The waving that is done in these establishments has a special character of its own, which can be recognised from afar – a sort of rigid, set, regular groove, very pronounced and so formal that it can be compared to the effect seen in wood carving. This arises from the fact that the new war-emergency female hairdressers, not having yet acquired the dexterity necessary for properly dressing the hair, simply use the hot iron for making parallel impressions on the hair. And that is quite sufficient to meet the wishes and requirements of this special class of customers who have not yet reached the stage when they can appreciate a true undulation, soft and serpentine.

In the upper circles it is quite the contrary. Those ladies who continue to use their own hair for their coiffure show themselves very particular in this matter, seeking only the very best undulation, with large, soft waves, in which the iron leaves no trace of breakage. Such clients have no regard for price, paying readily any sum up to twenty francs for the work of an expert who provides exactly what they require. But the ladies who have their own hair dressed are a diminishing quantity. Three-fourths, or perhaps four-fifths, to-day wear postiche, according to their age. Therefore the leading Parisian coiffeurs are specialists in postiche and their establishments are located in the centre of the city, whilst all the other ladies' hairdressers principally confine themselves to waving. If it should happen that they effect a sale of postiche, it is always a *postiche d'utilité* – that is to say, it is used to supplement the natural hair of the customer, which is insufficiently thick or too short.

In the case of the large posticheurs the circumstances are again different and distinct. They principally sell *postiche de luxe* and *de fantasie* for covering the natural hair that may have been cut, or which it may be desired to hide in order to acquire a different and stronger hair tint, or a prettier and more fashionable style of coiffure.

The point that remains is whether postiche de luxe entirely fulfils its mission, which is to provide complete and durable satisfaction to the client. Here I must draw a distinction. There are two categories of wearers of postiche: those who know the proper employment of false hair, because they have learnt it, or because they have used it for a long time; and those who wear postiche for the first time and who, not knowing its proper use, place it badly, fail to comb it or else comb it the wrong way, cut it, curl it with the iron or dye it themselves in order to alter it according to their own taste. The latter need guidance and assistance, and usually they gain knowledge at their own expense. The posticheur is not always in close and immediate touch with his client, and in spite of his advice and directions, he occasionally experiences an irritating visit from a lady who is consumed with anger and complaints, and who on examination he discovers is wearing her transformation the wrong way round!

But generally speaking the best postiche invariably gives satisfaction, for this industry has acquired in these days a degree of perfection which can scarcely be surpassed because it equals the highest natural qualities of artistic attractiveness. I do not think I exaggerate when I say that [the best] postiche, which allows of such instantaneous, complete, and characteristic transformations, is a notable production. The quality of hair is the finest that can be found, and the foundation is also very expertly executed by work girls who are paid twenty francs per day if they work on the premises of the posticheur, or who take sixty francs per piece if they do their work at home. Such a postiche is sold for from 400 to 500 francs (£16 to £20) in the prettiest up-to-date tints, and at much higher prices if the hair is grey or of rare colour.

December 1918: Developments in Bridal Coiffures

Having been present recently, either as coiffeur or simply as a spectator, at several grand Parisian weddings, I am able to submit descriptions and sketches of the headdresses that were worn. At first, the *toilettes* after the latest fashion – skirts extremely short and bodices very low at the neck – shocked me considerably. It seemed to me that there were three stages in life when one should respect recognised and conventional modes – I mean the ceremonies of (1) the first communion, (2) of marriage, and (3) of burial. It would seem,

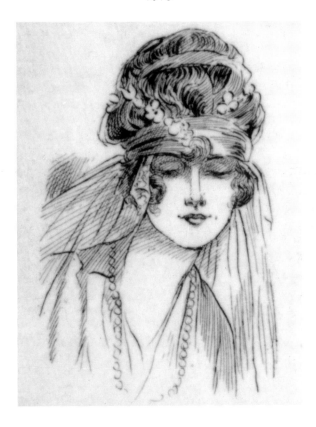

Figure 31. A bridal coiffure at one of the grand Parisian weddings. From *HWJS,*
December 1918.

however, that this view is no longer recognised, and I am compelled to admit
that I was in error, since at these functions, and especially in the case of
weddings and on occasions of deep mourning, Parisiennes wear white or
black but follow the very latest styles. In the case of joy as of anguish, *la
fantasie* triumphs absolutely.

Every imaginable fantasy is to-day permitted to the coiffeur. He need no
longer hamper himself with former scruples, but may boldly submit his
conceptions to public judgment, with the one condition of being in agreement
with the tastes of his client. I believe that the more these conceptions are
enterprising and original, the more charming will be the effects secured, and
the greater will be the reputation of the artist.

The ornaments of orange blossom have disappeared almost entirely. To-
day in their place small white roses are used, or tiny lilies, or even a number
of fancy artificial flowers in white satin or velvet, or white muslin, etc. A

good deal of embroidery is also used now. In any case these ornaments are no longer placed in the hair itself in the form of a diadem or cluster; they now are employed by way of wreaths, coronets or delicate garlands, and are placed above the veil in various ways. In view of the foregoing, I think it will be conceded that my opening remark as to the greatest fancy and latitude being now permitted was justified.

10

1919

January 1919: For the Victory Galas

The Great Victory will be followed by many grand receptions and galas, for which extensive preparations are being made in Paris. In fact, the official receptions have already commenced, and certain dressmaking and hair-dressing firms have benefited financially from them; but these houses, which are very well known and restricted in number, are almost entirely noted for the brilliance and lavish character of their productions. Such work is certainly profitable to the privileged circle who monopolise it, but it possesses only a passing interest for the great bulk of the public who, being usually younger, prefer novelty and originality.

The older and classical styles, which are those of the official world, have therefore little interest for the generality of coiffeurs, and especially for the bold, enterprising innovators, whose essential object must be to give satisfaction to the numerous devotees of Fashion – the young and very modern ladies of elegance whom the men of wealth dote over. Like the high-spirited horse that is fed on the best oats and which impatiently paws the earth when deprived of freedom, a large number of these elegant females, whom the sorrows of the war have not touched, have generated during the long period of restrictions an absorbing desire for show, amusement and pleasure. The greater portion of them, it is true, have never missed any opportunity which offered for giving full scope to their *coquetterie*, but they have exercised a certain restraint out of regard for general opinion. Henceforth they will be less inclined to recognise any such reserve and the happier conditions which now prevail will relieve them of any necessity for it. They can expend money and amuse themselves extravagantly in broad daylight.

In order to administer to their caprices the industries *de luxe* are working at high pressure. There is a veritable furore amongst the specialist costumiers in the production of the prettiest robes for evening wear; and in the same way great demand is being made on the coiffeurs and posticheurs who have built up reputations for taste and new ideas.

The artist posticheurs are successful because they make it possible and easy to transform very rapidly, and always to embellish the feminine head

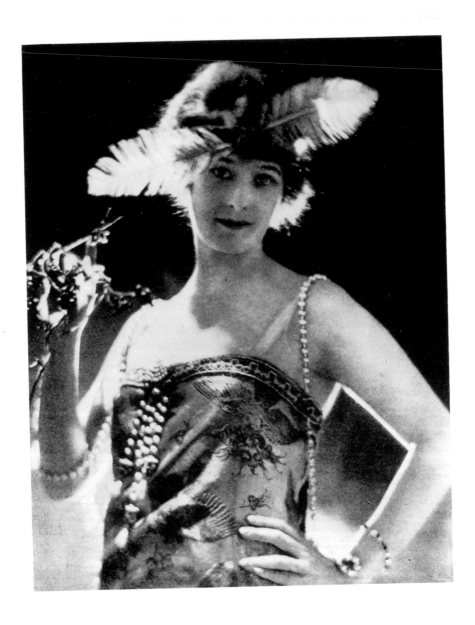

Figure 32. Flapper with a short, feathered coiffure. From *Vanity Fair*, March 1921.

with a new coiffure. In the case of a lady of position and elegance, to be able to secure quickly a better appearance is of the highest importance. The question of cost is relatively of no consequence, and is seldom a matter of serious consideration.

A second category comprises those who, under the title of *coiffeur des dames*, engage only in waving, bleaching, dyeing and the care of the hair. These experts take advantage of every opportunity to practise all kinds of ondulation and of tinting, instead of specialising in only one kind, one process or one preparation. And they achieve very considerable results from the point of view both of quantity of patronage and of profit. It is houses of this category which are now attracting many clients, who usually remain so long for attendance that they are served with tea, with bread and chocolate, until such time as the delicacies now prohibited are again obtainable. Wide experience is equally necessary in the cases of these men so that they may be able to decide what is requisite for each particular client and to achieve success where sometimes perhaps others have failed. For naturally, as in the practices of the leading physicians, cases of considerable difficulty are always encountered, which are submitted to the hair wavers or hair dyers at high fees because of their reputations for being clever in their particular branches. Once having established a reputation, they must never make a mistake. They therefore have heavy responsibilities, and it is but justice that financial return for their efforts should be proportionate.

February 1919: The Ornamentation of the High Coiffure

Speaking generally, it is invariably the high coiffure which meets with the greatest success in Paris; and in spite of rumours circulated from time to time, which lead some to suppose that a change of style has become desirable, no real indication has yet been given by the leading *élégantes* that there is any near rival to the high headdress, which adds to ladies' stature and imparts smartness. By gathering her hair on the crown, a lady frees her neck, which enhances the general effect of the line of the profile and gives a younger appearance.

For the high-style hairdressing, we in Paris are now perfectly organised; we know the mechanism from the foundation, and our supply houses, who are equally well equipped, assist by their useful co-operation. The necessary combs and barrettes and the great many other small articles and appliances for ornamentation are being produced in infinite variety. They are very easy in use, because we are all perfectly in accord in our aim – namely, the high coiffure.

All ladies who have fine heads of hair have not yet adopted the new whim of sacrificing same to the scissors. However, this freakish whim continues in Paris, and we shall be called upon to cut a number of heads of hair yet before it passes away. The more timid have about half cut off – to 25 or 30 centimètres; others, who are more numerous, want it cut to 15 or 20 centimètres; whilst the most audacious do not hesitate to wear the masculine coiffure. But all resort to curling or waving; it is the one thing which differentiates the last-named from the majority of men's heads. The last client that I had for permanent hair-waving had her hair cut so short that she gave the greatest possible difficulty. The base of the neck was almost bare, the clippers having been used, and around the ears the hair had been cut with the scissors by a gent's hairdresser. On the top of the head and at the crown the length of the tresses was no more than six or seven centimètres. The result before the final shampoo was a pretty curl to each strand of hair. After the shampoo and careful putting into pli, a magnificent series of waves was secured, just like the head of a young man who has a very nice and regular natural wave.

From my experience in this case I have arrived at the conclusion that it is possible, with the exercise of the necessary care and the expenditure of time, to execute permanent waving on the male head as well as on women's hair. I make this statement for the enlightenment of those of my Trade colleagues who would not have ventured to undertake such a task, and in order to show an extension of the possibilities of permanent waving, which has come into such great prominence of late.

The Americans are content to have their straight hair transformed into curly hair by the usual process of permanent waving; generally they do not attach importance to the form of the curl, because they look merely for a practical result. But the Parisiennes can discern the better appearance which is obtainable from very large waves, which they arrange admirably in the dressing of their usual coiffure. It is consequently very difficult to persuade them to accept the small, single waves that are obtained with the curlers of one thickness that are now made and sold by the manufacturers of permanent waving outfits. This difficulty would not arise if attention was paid to so simple a detail.

March 1919: Progress in Permanent Hair-waving

When about to be shampooed, the hair of my lady, which is naturally frizzy, bears a resemblance to astrakhan. That is to say, that it is much too curly. But whilst still wet it is well combed, backwards, and then pushed back with the comb, when fine waves are formed, which remain until the next shampoo.

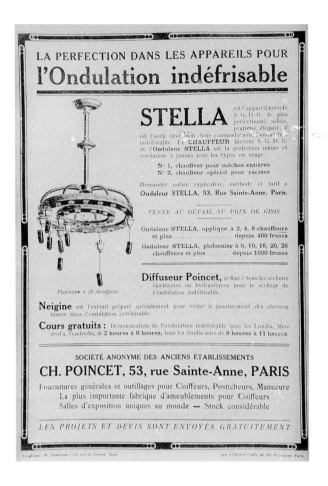

Figure 33. 'L'Ondulation indéfrisable' – advertisement for the permanent-wave machine, 'Stella'. From *La Coiffure de Paris*, 1922.

On examining this natural undulation, so soft and harmonious, I often think that it was to some such waves that the illustrious Marcel owed the inspiration which prompted him to create his immortal method. As with all the greatest artists, he could produce nothing better than a perfect imitation of one of the prettiest works of Nature. And it is accomplished with just a simple iron. But, then, why is it that not nearly all of those who use identically similar irons achieve the same result? Ah! Whilst it is true that a good instrument is necessary, it is equally true that experience and expertness are also requisite.

I hope I shall be pardoned for this somewhat abstract preamble, but I could not forget the invention of Marcel when thinking of permanent waving, because without the former the latter would never have existed. However, it does exist and has progressed, and it will certainly advance a good deal more yet.

Amongst the makers of the outfits and appliances for producing permanent waving, and who advertise in the English and American journals the superiority and advantages of their machines, several have already informed me that they are willing to come to Paris in order to demonstrate the improvements which they have made in this up-to-date treatment of the hair. Already one has visited Paris and has given an extremely interesting demonstration. That is M. Eugène of London, whose apparatus is really perfect, but in the handling of which competency and expertness are very necessary.

The entire hair, divided into thirty strands, was curled twice and then well shampooed, afterwards being very cleverly put into pli, and finally dried. The complete operation took about three hours. Then for something like an hour the hair was closely examined and handled by each of the 250 or 300 persons present, who one after the other subsequently put questions and queries to the demonstrator, and also the model. The demonstration was given at one of the public schools of hairdressing, before male and female hairdressers of all grades, and including a certain number from outside Paris.

Personally I noted with pleasure the progress that has been made in a system that I employed here some ten years ago. First, a notable reduction in the size of the heaters, with consequently the use of less currency and therefore less expense. The result, too, was more elegant. There was an entire absence of steam on the head, even when working with fifteen or thirty heaters at one time, thus obviating the need for fans and other generators of cold air. The reduction in the time occupied in the execution was considerable, since a half, three-quarters, or even the whole strand of hair could be heated at one time. It is possible to regulate the heater so that the heat is applied longer to the roots (which are always harder to curl) than to the points. A further advantage is that the intensity of the wave can be adjusted with the combination heater, and the size of all the waves regulated by the conical bigoudi which is used. Again, the bigoudi can be worked up quite close to the head, and it is possible for a lady to tighten it on the strand of hair at will. The steaming pad is a very clean and practical appliance. Nevertheless there may be a little complication caused by the many ends of string, and much care, precaution and personal judgment are necessary, [in view of] the risk of curling like a poodle dog a head of hair which required only a few large and soft waves.

April 1919: Fashionable Parisian Ladies' Attempt to Alter Hairdressing Styles

The various fetes which are in course of preparation in Paris are creating business for all engaged in the trades *de luxe*, including those who are labouring for Art, and even a large number of reputed artists. The big jewellers are designing sensationally conspicuous ornaments, amongst which may be mentioned some splendid diamond diadems for headdress wear – the diamonds being varied with pearls and fine sparkling stones of different colours.

In order that such gems may be well displayed upon the heads of the little Queens of Fashion, light and cleverly made postiche becomes necessary in the form of nice soft hair, *mousse d'or*, jet-black curls, as the poets say, shining and vaporous waves over auburn locks, with the reflections of pale red mahogany or copper coloured hues. All this can be obtained artificially when Nature refuses, thanks to the skill and professional ingenuity of the modern coiffeur.

At the present moment, fashionable ladies are making audacious efforts to rid themselves of a fashion (the enveloping style) which has lasted ten years at least in one form or another. This is far too long for a feminine fashion. It happens, therefore, that some ladies are torturing themselves so much that their hair breaks and assumes of its own accord a more modern aspect; and should the hair resist all sorts of torture, it is cut off, thus bringing about the longed for radical change.

Sometimes, however, these undisciplined curls become unruly, and their frizzy appearance assumes exaggerated proportions. The dishevelled state of her hair alarms the coquette, who, losing patience, seizes a ribbon or a lock of long straight hair and encircles it around the head. In this way the lady quickly obtains a charming coiffure, which, no doubt, soon becomes general amongst her circle of friends, who find in it the expression of a new fashion.

[Some women] decorate their hair with very pretty waves; others take advantage of an abundance of hirsute growth by massing their coque chignon on top. But the latter are criticised and ironically termed '*bourgeoises*' by other ladies who find the high coiffure too 'common' and vulgar, since factory lasses and suburbanites have adopted this fashion.

It comes about, therefore, that a notable portion of fashionable ladies do not care to cut their hair, and that they do not approve of the high chignon. For these people there remain two equally classical styles: either the back headdress with the ends of the hair arranged in different ways on the nape of the neck, or the style worn by the little typists in Paris, which is obtained by rolling the plait over the ears after the form of a snail.

May 1919: The Decline of Short Hair

The fashion of short hair for ladies has become so general in Paris, that all the French papers, even the most serious, are dealing with the question at the present time. Articles are appearing one after the other and are multiplying in number almost everywhere, whilst the illustrated magazines are presenting an abundance of coiffures showing the hair cut short, and all sorts of caricatures on the same subject. Artists have become so used to the fashion that they are embodying it in all their sketches, with the result that various trade catalogues display figures with the hair cut in this way.

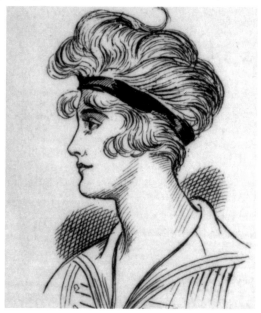

Figure 34. A fashionable short hairstyle, one of the models 'most characteristic at . . . the shops of the most up-to-date of ladies' hairdressers'. From *HWJS*, May 1919.

According to an article which I have seen in the *Daily Mail* [a British newspaper], it is clear that almost the same fashion is in vogue in London, and nearly everywhere else. Only, it is in Paris and principally in the eccentric quarter of Montmartre, that these coiffures should be seen! I should never have supposed that short cut hair would lend itself to such a large variety of fancy head-dresses. Ladies with dark hair generally adopt the sea-lion style of coiffure, with large pointed, heavy and shiny locks, or a few large rolls right at the extremities. Some wear their hair all frizzed like poodles and dressed exceptionally high; others only frizz the ends of the hair and dress all the remainder straight and flat. In a word, the majority of these women, with their overdone make-up and peculiar head-dresses, look more like clowns straight from the circus that any category of female.

It must not be supposed that only the young and frivolous have taken to this fashion; to-day coiffures of short hair and short postiche may be seen in every circle, even amongst the upper ten, and amongst certainly elderly ladies with light grey hair. By the bye, in a certain house where the husband has perforce to wear a wig and the wife, to satisfy her fancy, wears one too, the servant handed to her master in mistake the short wig meant for his wife!

The first question which the journalists put to me is this: 'Where does this fashion come from?' *Eh, parbleu*, it comes from the need of a change which has coincided with the events taking place in Russia, that's all. All the great political revolutions have brought about an upheaval in fashions and notably as regards ladies' hair. Read history: The coiffure *à la Titus* caused a furore amongst the French when the 18th century sank in a sea of blood. Briefly, the short coiffures appeared after the *Terreur*, Notre Dame de Thermidor had short hair, and the beautiful ladies who escaped the guillotine wore their hair '*à la victime*.'

And when will this style take on again? This will be when people begin to speak of the events in Russia, of Bolshevism and the Red Terror. A member of our trade, who came from Russia about 18 months ago, has done the cutting of more ladies' hair in Paris than all the other coiffeurs put together.

Again, short hair is a sign of the times. The woman who works becomes manly; she has no time to care for her coiffure, being deprived of her former leisure. There is also another reason: feminism is rising, carrying with it principles which evoke equality of the sexes. Is not woman's long hair a sign of servitude? Short hair typifies a programme of franchise, as we are given to understand, when a wise woman orders her hair to be cut and dressed *à l'indépendance*.

Who knows but that in their patriotism the women of the allied nations have not wished to improve the German philosopher Schopenhauer, who said that woman was a being who had 'short ideas and long hair.'

In reality, it is only a passing fashion, and one which is already beginning to pass, for the majority of those who adopted it a year or two ago are now tired of and disgusted with it.

June 1919: Ribbon as Ornament for the Hair

Everybody knows how fashionable strands of velvet and other material are at the moment for binding round the coiffure and forehead.

Ribbons are essentially articles which come within the realm of the drapery establishments, and the directors of these concerns have seized the opportunity to promote an enormous propaganda on the subject. They have instructed their artists to add ribbons to the headdresses of all the figures which they sketch both for catalogue and fashion papers. The aid of producers of cinematograph films have likewise been enlisted in this matter, so that the public may be presented as often as possible with coiffures displaying ribbons.

The result of all this propaganda is that nowadays in Paris even the meanest midinette [office-girl or shop-girl] or milliner's assistant sports her little bit of ribbon. And, moreover, in spite of the constantly rising prices, shops are daily selling miles of velvet and other kinds of ribbon.

The beautiful ornaments which we carefully composed every season and afterwards placed so tastefully in the coiffure now remain in their boxes, or else fade away in the shop windows, whilst clients ask the hairdresser to place in their hair 'the little thing which they picked up' when passing by such and such a shop. Certain artists, it is true, refuse point blank to insert anything which does not come from their own shop, but the general run of hairdressers accede to the request. In any case, there is nothing to prevent the client from posing the ribbon herself. It is so simple!

July 1919: Voluptuousness Rampant

In face of the unexampled and extraordinary habits of luxury which are in evidence in Paris, at the present time, where is the individual in the Hair-dressing Trade who has sufficient psychology to discover the influences connecting the feminine toilette with the great worldly social upheavals?

There has not been, since the great French Revolution, any event to be compared with the cataclysm which has just come to an end; and it is strange to reflect that the two epochs have had a similar influence on ladies' toilette. After the Reign of Terror, the modes were particularly voluptuous. The dainty females who escaped the guillotine at that period dressed – or rather deshabilled – themselves in the fashion of the ancients; clothed in very low cut robes, their coquetry went so far as to cause them to expose the lovely curves of their stockingless legs, and the sculptural shape of their feet, disclosing the toes ornamented with rings. The veils of the *Merveilleuses*[1] of the Directoire period could not pass for clothes; they were 'threaded wind,'

---

1. The provocatively clad young women of the French Revolution in the period following the fall of Robespierre in July 1794.

as a wit of that time remarked. After Waterloo our great grandmothers wrapped themselves in damp muslin robes so that in the process of drying, the folds clung more voluptuously to the form of the body.

To-day, after the Gothas and Berthas,[2] after the terrible anguish of the war, we move again amongst the fashions of the ancients. Ladies reveal their shoulders; corsets have, so to speak, disappeared; and the habit of applying a depilatory beneath the arms has been acquired. The dispensers of depilatories and the manufacturers of make-up are in fact, doing a roaring business.

Again, our fashionable ladies have shortened their skirts to an exaggerated extent; thus showing their calves enclosed in veritable spider's webbed stockings.

But even this is insufficient. On the Auteuil Race Course recently, a group of coquettes caused a considerable sensation on account of their invisible stockings. 'What are they made of?' wondered the other envious ladies, 'they are finer than silk.' In the end they solved the problem. Our new 'Merveilleuses' simply had bare legs, like their ancestors of the Directoire period. In reality their calves were covered with make-up, similar to their faces. Since then, bare legs are to be seen everywhere.

Safety razors now have a place in almost every lady's toilet cabinet, being used after bathing to embellish the legs. A whole category of specialists is being organised at the moment to go from house to house for the purpose of massaging and making-up ladies' legs.

When we attend to dress the hair of ladies who so far have not indulged in outdoor exercise with their nether limbs clothed in nakedness, we find them in pyjamas, their hair cut short, smoking cigarettes and looking very much like little boys escaped from college. Most of the ladies have their necks shaved, especially during the warm weather; then they flatly wave the remainder of their hair, except for one lock at each side, which hangs in curls or large waves. This style is called the 'Dog's Ear' coiffure. The object of this special form of headdress is to show a little hair framing the visage under hats which reach down to the eyes in front and cover the nape of the neck at the back.

In any case, the head-dress ornaments, for evening wear, follow the luxuriousness of the toilet, which is very pronounced. Diamond bands, materials of gold, magnificent feathers and combs are to be seen everywhere.

---

2. The reference is to German artillery pieces.

August 1919: Coiffures and Postiche Worn by Middle-class Parisiennes

Nowadays waving has penetrated everywhere, and ladies' hairdressers may consequently be found in every part of our capital, several in each provincial town, and at least one in every village.

There is no doubt that this popularity is due to the famous invention of the Marcel, for the majority of these ladies' hairdressers do not know how to dress the hair and are only competent in waving.

However, waving brings along the lady clients, who really teach hairdressers their trade by forcing them to shampoo and dye their hair, to sell and pose pieces of postiche. Thus, with patience and a desire to succeed, practice makes perfect. Eventually the barber's shop develops into a veritable ladies' hairdressing establishment.

Of the three-thousand hairdressing establishments which exist in Paris, there are to-day hardly two hundred which do simply haircutting and shaving; all the others cover waving and other work connected with it. Twenty years ago, things were quite different; ladies' hands were then very scarce. At the present time at least one wax figure may be seen in the window of any shop where waving is practised, and not infrequently several are on view. The manufacture and production of wax figures has greatly increased during the last twenty years. The Parisian coiffeurs alone possess about ten thousand, not to mention the corset makers, modistes, perfume houses, comb merchants, etc., etc. The big drapery firms possess between four and five hundred each. In short, these wax figures total approximately 50,000 in Paris alone. This represents an average of 10,000,000 in France.

And the remarkable part of all this is that nearly every one of these busts is dressed in very much the same style. Of course, these figures have no hair, and are dressed by means of postiche. But even those which still have hair implanted in the war are all dressed in similar style. I have tried to ascertain if all these coiffeurs have studied in the same school and under the same instructor. But, no! The reason appears to be that the majority do not know how to make postiche, and that in order to sell all the hair they are asked for, they buy ready-made postiche from trade houses, who are at the moment all turning out the same model. It seems to be a rather convenient idea, too, for this postiche (big, enveloping style) can be bought and sold like a hat or any other commercial commodity.

At the establishments of the grands maîtres posticheurs, who create and manufacture very fine models with superior quality hair, the fashionable ladies have to wait several days, sometimes weeks, even months, and then pay an exceedingly high price. This they are prepared to do, simply because they have the means and insist on having the very best in every case.

The middle-class ladies, however, are more numerous and much less exacting, with the result that good business can be done in copied models manufactured by the hundred. In all the large drapery establishments, perfumery and hairdressing shops these goods are freely sold.

September 1919: Toilets, Coiffures and Head Ornaments for Next Season

I referred to feminine fashions in the *Supplement* for July, and particularly to the voluptuous modes shown at the theatre, in a play called 'Amoureuse,' by a beautiful and talented actress, named Mlle. Ventura.

In the second act of this play, Mlle. Ventura wore a delicious dress which created a great sensation. Her shoulders, in their beautiful bareness, displayed the sweetness of her bust to the fullest advantage. As much of the front part of the figure was left uncovered as the physical formation – that is to say, of a well-made woman – would allow, whilst the back was uncovered in an impeccable drop to the curve of the back. It was elegant, captivating and daringly *chic*. Chrysis of old could not have imagined a more fitting fashion. This lovely dress, so short that it showed the knees at the slightest movement of the silken fringes which terminated it, has since been reproduced and even exaggerated by certain fashionable females who parade the streets with bare arms, bare legs and short hair, frizzed like little school boys.

At all the holiday resorts there are multitudes of Parisiennes, doubly *décolletées*, who daily use depilatories and beauty aids on every visible part of their beautiful bodies. The coiffeurs-saisonniers (hairdressers doing a season trade) have done brilliant business in all this kind of speciality, frizzing short hair and disposing of natural wavy postiche when indignant 'hubbies' could no longer tolerate their wives with such short crops.

Whilst the season hands have been making money, those who did not leave Paris have profited by the slack season in putting their shops into good trim and devising new models in postiche or ornaments for the coming season. M. Perrin, the new President of the Institut des Coiffeurs de Dames de France, wanted to take advantage of the many meetings which have been held in Paris on the subject of the 48 hour week[3] (definitely adopted by the ladies' hairdressers) to restart the séance of former times, when ideas were exchanged

3. Soon after the war, the French legislated a 48-hour work week, at least in principle, for all French employees.

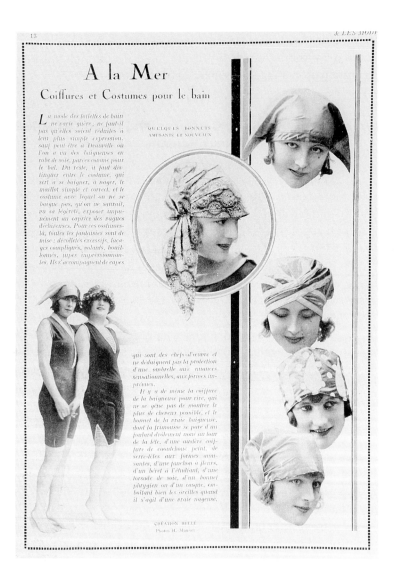

Figure 35. 'A la Mer' – coiffures and swimsuits at the seaside resorts. From *La Coiffure de Paris*, 1922.

on the subject of hairdressing fashions. Personally I prefer these kind of consultations and mutual understandings to the cold decisions laid down by the official fashion committee. In the course of the last few meetings it was agreed, without obligation on anybody, that the fashion should continue *high*, except that instead of having the prominence formed by the chignon quite on top of the head, it should be arranged just a little to the rear.

I have also taken several sketches of head ornaments in our various *salles de spectacles* [theatres]. [In the first] the feathers appear to come out of the ears, and their horizontal position makes them a source of annoyance to people sitting next to the wearer. [The second] represents a sort of ornament which also caused me no little surprise, for the feather is placed in a fashion which is contrary to the usual custom. This is a style adopted by fashionable ladies who, frankly would appear ridiculous were they not so pretty. But when people are in possession of the advantages of youth and beauty, everything is permissible. And I perceive that nobody cares a rap.

October 1919: Is Fashion Changing

A Parisian journal has just made the sensational announcement that the 'low' head-dress is the fashion. This has caused some trouble to the coiffeurs, whose daily experience proves (1) that the low head-dress is not fashionable; (2) that if they popularised the low chignon, with the present style of front, coiffeurs would have to stop working up and selling postiche. The eight-hour day would then be too long for dealing with the work which this style of head-dress would produce.

Those who understand better the needs of a trade and take an interest in its requirements and interests think less of astonishing than of serving the profession. For our own part, we cannot admit that the low coiffure is fashionable, for this is not the truth. Neither can we ask our readers to push this low coiffure, because we know as practical people that this style of hairdressing would not be advantageous at this moment of relative simplicity. So long as hats descend in front over the eyes and extend at the back to the neck, and so long as headgear is of the narrow kind, compelling us to flatten the coiffure all round the head, there will be no advantage in hairdressers favouring such a radical change.

Now that Marcel waving has slowly brought lady customers back to our saloons and that multitudes of assistants, both male and female, gain a livelihood from practising this speciality, it behoves us to be very careful not to allow any ill-thought-out caprice to spoil the section of our industry which supplies bread to so many families.

November 1919: Eclecticism in Modern Ladies' Hairdressing

The greatest eclecticism is reigning at the moment in ladies' hairdressing. During the holiday season at Trouville-Deauville, and the autumnal season at Biarritz, where the fashionable folk of all countries disport themselves, about ten styles of hairdressing were to be noticed, the difference between them being about as marked as that which exists between the sun and the moon. With their long hair, half-long or short hair, or extremely short hair, some ladies emerged triumphant with entirely straight tresses; others with very curly locks, others with widely-waved or medium-waved hair; either with clearly defined large curls, or else ordinary combed out curls. There were high, medium and low coiffures to be seen; coiffures in which the front hair was drawn back so as to uncover the whole forehead, and others, on the contrary, where the forehead was quite hidden by flat fringes or very large puffs. All these styles met with approval and were considered charming. [In] Paris just now neat, regular and quiet styles are to be seen, obtained with pretty pieces of postiche, extremely wide and softly waves; also electrically waved hair can be seen, embelished with gold and silver ribbon. Yes, permanent hair waving is beginning to catch on in Paris, and in its own characteristic way is capable of very pretty effects when it is executed by an experienced assistant.

[The eminent coiffeur] M. Jourliac claims that really fashionable ladies are at present disgusted with the ugly and too rigid style of waving which is everywhere done very cheaply and worn by servant girls and factory hands. They are clamouring for a radical change and have tried the mode of cut hair. Immediately afterwards short hair was to be seen all over the city and even among the servant girls and factory hands. Only one way, therefore, is left to fashionable ladies to distinguish themselves, and that is to wear straight, or almost straight hair.

December 1919: Lowering the Chignon

The fashionable clients are now [back] in Paris, where luxury is rife and money is freely spent. I have been to the races, the theatres, and also to the very numerous dancing establishments where I might, with a bit of luck, perceive some new headdresses. Like my confrères who usually take season places, I have seen very few low coiffures.

Besides these low headdresses I perceived others which are not worth describing, for they would occasion us much more harm than good. But, fortunately, I have also seen a few very pretty and gorgeous high and half-high coiffures, some dressed with magnificent modern postiche, and others with natural hair permanently waved. This permanent waving, which the Parisiennes would not have at any price when presented in its natural form, now interests them enormously. There is already a large number of fashionable ladies here who have had their hair waved with electrical appliances and who come back to the coiffeur every week to have it water waved. As a rule ten francs is charged for this service, but some artistes obtain higher prices still. This source of income is a fortunate one, which those who were not in favour of the system had not foreseen, when in their systematic hostility they sought to spread the rumour that once they had their hair electrically waved clients would return to the hairdresser no more. Not only do they return every week, but on average they have their hair re-waved every six months.

Well, it is being agreed that we take ten francs per curler – that is to say, 300 to 500 francs for an entire head – it will not be difficult to work out the amount spent by clients in the shop of those progressive hairdressers who, instead of decrying this process, were amongst the first to adopt it. I will not dwell on the handsome tips which these clients present to the employees, and the large sales which may be made to ladies who spend such sums of money on nothing but hair-waving. All the big vedettes of the cinemas and theatres, numbers of *grandes dames du monde*, and all the 'new rich' are having recourse to this process of hair-waving.

War-time simplicity is commencing to disappear and make way for *grande coquetterie* and luxury, in spite of the unheard-of-prices of everything. Money is circulating more quickly than has been the case for a long, long time.

11

1920

January 1920: Public Hairdressing Exhibition in Paris

The public, especially the ladies, are always easily interested in everything affecting their coquetry, and more rightly so in hairdressers' beauty products, which are not only luxurious but often very necessary for purposes of hygiene and cleanliness.

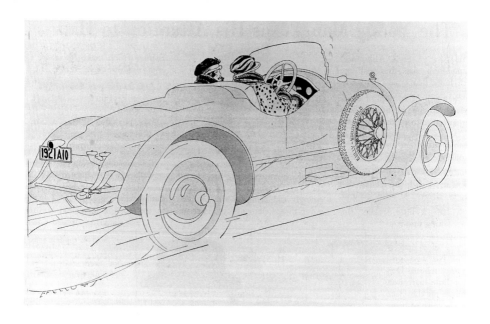

Figure 36. A cliché of the sporty young socialite of the postwar years – two elegant young women out motoring. From *Vanity Fair*, February 1921.

Unfortunately, up to the present time, owing to the open-door system, our profession has been overcrowded with a mass of indigence which, instead of helping, has kept us down to the level of the small trades. The efforts of the intelligent have always been met with apathy, and consequently have failed to achieve anything big. This means that the public have been unable to learn sufficient as regards the products of the *coiffeur*, who has, therefore, lost a large part of his trade.

However, in the seventeenth century even, a *coiffeur* exhibited at the big fairs, a whole series of plaster busts, the heads of which were dressed after the fashion of the day, or rather in the various styles which were worn by the different classes of society. In the eighteenth century there were more than one *coiffeur de dames* who had gained renown, and the principal amongst them paid young ladies to parade the grand boulevards with their hair dressed in the latest *mode*. In the evenings other ladies were paid to exhibit themselves at the most popular theatrical performances with a view to advertising other styles of *coiffures*. As may be imagined, these exhibitions cost quite a lot of money, but were nevertheless beneficial to the whole Trade.

At the Universal Exhibitions of Paris in 1889 and 1900 and even at the National Exhibitions between these two dates, there were at Paris some memorable displays of wax figures which, *coiffed* and draped regardless of expense, scored a great success amongst the fashionable public. Under the auspices of the Académie de Coiffure numerous ladies' hairdressers came to an agreement (no small achievement) under which they jointly put forth considerable efforts which naturally brought very appreciable results.

[Today, on the contrary] pride and selfishness are to be found among all the big men; each one maintains his claim to being the sole creator of fashion; whilst among the small men, who are in the majority, indifference and hopeless apathy are to be observed.

These small men are waiting to see what the big men are going to do, and the latter are not doing anything much on account of the rivalry and jealousy which exists amongst them. In short, each one is on the look out for himself, but no one is prepared to give anything away.

An individual who was, no doubt, filled with good intentions, but ignorant of the difficulties of organisation, attempted recently to hold a hairdressing exhibition for the public. He had received written promises of help from thirty committees. At the moment of putting his plans into operation, however, there was not a single one willing to render assistance. Everybody begged to be excused, and in consequence the idea had to fall through.

February 1920: The Day of 'Modern' Ideas and Extravagance

It is evident that after-war is even greater than pre-war extravagance. And the more it is talked about, the more apparently it continues. Such is the power of advertisement – and there are eminently contagious example of it.

In Paris there are some young ladies of perfect education and unquestionable moral qualities who exist unnoticed, and who will have difficulty in marrying because they have not adopted the risky modern style; because they do not display their present-day coquetry and lack of constraint.

There are likewise in Paris some coiffeurs of a certain age who have not the courage to move with the times and who are slowly losing their livelihood by having their trade taken from them. These tradesmen are the ones who do not mix with their confrères and who do not take sufficient interest in affairs outside their own doors. Confined to their shops, with their old-fashioned methods, they are forced to recognise, though slowly, that their work does not attract; yet they refuse to change their out-of-date methods and then complain of hard times; they complain of the hardness of fate or else bemoan that the public of to-day have no taste and do not appreciate real elegance.

In our profession, which deals with fashion and luxuries, one must either move on or get out. A coiffeur must be all eyes and ears, quick to make profit out of all he sees and hears. The personal taste of the hairdresser must always bow before that of his client shows how it should be done; and if she is confronted with obstinacy and does not receive satisfaction, she can very easily carry her money elsewhere. Even the most faithful and amiable clients, those who swear they could never do without us, finish by leaving us on the most slender excuse. Their oaths of fidelity are rather like oaths of lovers or the inebriated – very superficial, and disperse as soon as they leave the lips.

What, then, is the proper course of action? Pay attention! Sell what sells, do what is done and wear what is worn. Luxury triumphs; then let us adopt luxury. Very expensive perfumes, gold-mounted vaporisers and all articles *de luxe* are the readiest sold goods at the present time.

The styles of coiffure are of the most audacious description; the ornaments and combs are of the most expensive variety. And Paris coiffeurs are also making money from the sale of all kinds of hand-bags, jewellery, toilet necessaries and leather goods.

The question of money and price is not even mentioned. There is plenty of money about; everybody has got money and everybody is spending it. And, though he be an artiste, the coiffeur is before all a business man and like others he is profiting by the prevailing circumstances.

March 1920: The Menace of Chinese Hairdressing Styles

Hairdressers never agree when it is a question of creating and pushing a fashion, because each individual is too anxious for his own taste and interests to come out on top. But, on the other hand, in the event of a fashion being suddenly sprung upon the Trade by the public, all the hairdressers meet and knock their heads together like sheep at the approach of the storm.

This is what has just happened. Chinese fashions, which at the present moment have so much influence on French fashions in furnishing, decorating, and even ladies' clothes, have already invaded everywhere, from the top to the bottom of our houses, theatres, and our modern illustrated papers. The Chinese fashions exercise their influence on our manners, our customs and our gestures; they have captivated the manufacturers of cloths and boots; even artists in decoration, and all productions of luxury, ornamentation and coquetry have fallen under their influence. Only one thing escaped for a time, and that was the coiffure. But that could not last.

In order to be right up to date, several actresses – and not the least notorious amongst them – who had already dressed and made themselves up in the Chinese style, took it into their heads to dress their hair in the Chinese fashion which they did in the most exaggerated manner, drawing, smoothing and fixing their hair flatly so that it appeared as if it were painted on a bald head, paint actually being used to design the sharp points on the temples and forehead. Thus disfigured, these actresses showed themselves in various places for a few evenings – with great courage, it must be admitted, for the most polite spectators commenced to murmur, whilst others pelted them with bad apples and rotten oranges. Now they limit their attendances to private and intimate receptions. But even these few public exhibitions were sufficient to spread ribald rumours amongst our lady customers. Some believe it was a kind of black velvet bonnet; everywhere the rumour raged that neither waving, postiche, nor head ornaments were being worn – nothing, in fact, but the smoothest possible hair. Some clients cancelled orders for postiche which had been in hand for a long time and could not be executed through lack of lady boardworkers.[1]

Just imagine the immediate effect of all this on the hairdressing fraternity who believed themselves hopelessly lost. Then something happened which recalled the first days of the War. All the hairdressers formed a brotherhood – the opulent, casting aside their habitual pride, uniting with their humbler brethren and soliciting help in combating this new fashion, this accursed Chinese mode which was to be the ruin of the profession in general and of

1. Workers who weave the postiche.

hairdressers in particular. They declared themselves ready to meet all expenses and take all the necessary steps as regards the Trade papers and illustrated magazines in order that such a fashion might not become general. The various societies and groups also held meetings and proceeded hand in hand to elaborate schemes for the Trade's defence. Arrangements were made for the bad Chinese styles to be immediately met by a profusion of really nice samples of hairdressing.

This system of publicity seems to be achieving excellent results, for the Chinese fashions have almost disappeared. But we have had a narrow escape. If this incident has the effect of bringing the Trade to a definite understanding between themselves the Chinese fashions will have achieved some useful purpose.

April 1920: The Ornamentation of the Coiffure

Formerly, when far fewer hairdressers were in existence and the ornaments for decorating ladies' coiffures were regulated by the age, social rank and style of each client, professional tuition was not to be obtained either by hook or crook. The apprentice coiffeur who set out to master ladies' hairdressing had to commence by making postiche, which was, and will always remain, the fundamental basis of our profession; then after a long experience of handling raw hair, he was instructed in the hygienic and technical aspects of living hair: cleaning the head, brushing, combing, applying lotions, pomades, powders, dyes, etc.

It was whilst learning these two stages that the apprentice became experienced and the clientèle gradually gained confidence in him. During this time he was slowly shown, on a practice block, the elementary rudiments of hairdressing. Then when the student had displayed sufficient aptitude he was allowed to start curling hair and to execute simple *coiffures de ville* – to assist the employer by passing him pins and helping in his artistic work.

This method of beginning at the commencement was infinitely more logical and produced much better results than the present-day procedure whereby tuition is given as quickly as possible in one branch only, which is at once and indefinitely exploited for all it is worth. The old system limited competition, whilst the later one fosters it and causes the working prices to fall. The modern coiffeur does not retain his clientèle for long, because his work is that of a specialist and not that of an artist. By specialising, he forces his clientèle to seek other specialists, and in this way the sale trade slips away from his fingers. The coiffeur of former times, on the other hand, retained his clients for himself by supplying every article used in the profession. As a rule, he made his own perfumery and toilet preparations, which he applied to the face and hands; oils, pomades and dyes for the hair; likewise, he manufactured all the postiche and ornaments necessary for his coiffures. As a result, there was more harmony in his creations and more profit in his business.

Nowadays the coiffeur does not dress the hair, in the strict sense of the word, and consequently, he has no opportunity to sell many hair ornaments. On many occasions, indeed, he is obliged to pose ornaments which have been purchased elsewhere, ornaments which are not at all suitable for certain kinds of coiffures, but are placed on all styles of headdresses and are removed at will.

In Paris, ladies have a thousand and one opportunities for evening wear and spend unheard of sums on their toilette and trinkets. I have noted numerous interesting facts during the brilliant Opera Season. Apart from the detestable Chinese style, which spoils the average physiognomy, I rather enjoyed the Egyptian style of dressing, with its coiffures of Cleopatra and the priestess of Isis, whose little false plaits gave our Parisian ladies the hieratic air of the trouble idols of ancient Egypt. The need for freedom, which is passing since the War, still keeps triumphant the boyish type of headdresses amongst those who have sacrificed their hair; the Tituses, Ninons, Jeannes d'Arc, with more or less curled hair, resort for evening wear to golden scarves, which they place like turbans around their heads; there are some, even, who still keep their Rasputin coiffures, with hair cut, falling on to the neck, uncurled, with a plain ribbon tied around.

There are many plumes, both falling and rampant, as if growing out of the ears, sometimes standing straight up at the back or protruding like fans. Beautiful decorated combs, rings, jewelled diadems alternate with rich embroidered material. Large brilliant diadems costing four or five hundred francs are no longer a rarity. Coloured stoned of unusual size are set with diamonds on headbands from under which electrically craped hair escapes. Pampille diadems at the side, rings and spheres of jade and jet, accompanied by a paradise plume lying on the shoulder, are the crowning glory of the fairly high blonde coiffures.

May 1920: A Form of Hairdressing which Pleases Everybody

At the present time the Grecian style of hairdressing is meeting with the approval of everybody, and is being adopted in some degree everywhere. It must be recognised that this ancient fashion lends itself to thousands of variations of elegant simplicity, and that if throughout the ages it has frequently been in vogue, the reason is because it responds so truly to our conceptions of beauty. Each epoch, it is true, brings some modifications of detail; we, for example, have added decoration in the form of Marcel waving. But on each occasion that the caprices of Fashion demanded relatively less voluminous coiffures recourse had to be had to ancient Greece, which possessed the most beautiful style which has ever existed.

[One version of the Grecian style] is a new attempt, which may be qualified as heroic, recently made in Paris by the Maison Emile et Cie., with a view to revivifying the profitable mode of curls on the neck. Whilst fully recognising the fine intention which has prompted our excellent *confrère* and friend M. Gaston Boudou,[2] we predict that he will experience a check as radical as it is complete. At the present time clients will not have curls on the neck and still less on the shoulders; they like the nape of the neck to feel free, whatever the coiffure. For ten years or more Trade leaders have worn themselves out in attempts similar to that referred to, actuated by the view that the interests of the Trade lie in the return of hanging curls. Some have displayed these in their show windows, and others have published them in the great illustrated papers; others, again, have attempted to introduce them into theatrical circles; some braving the ridicule evoked, have displayed them in their school demonstrations; all have endeavoured to sell them to their undecided clients. Wasted trouble! Fashionable ladies will not muffle themselves with these hanging curls, so much praised by the Trade. They obstinately refuse to cover up their necks.

When high collars were in fashion, ladies' hairdressers appreciated that it was difficult to push low chignons and falling curls so long as the corsages were not cut low. But of latter days they have been simply throwing money away, for these collars have died out of fashion; on the other hand, never has so much *décolletage* been witnessed as nowadays. The nape of the neck is now uncovered, but hanging curls have not come into vogue again; and fashionable ladies, for their part, are in no hurry to encumber themselves uselessly.

June 1920: Century-old Hairdressing to be Revived

This is the time of year when the young boys and girls of France take their first Communion – the girls in their traditional white robes, with a white

---

2. Boudou, whose salon occupied Robespierre's former apartments on the rue Saint-Honoré, was also the inventor of the first French permanent-wave machine, the Gallia.

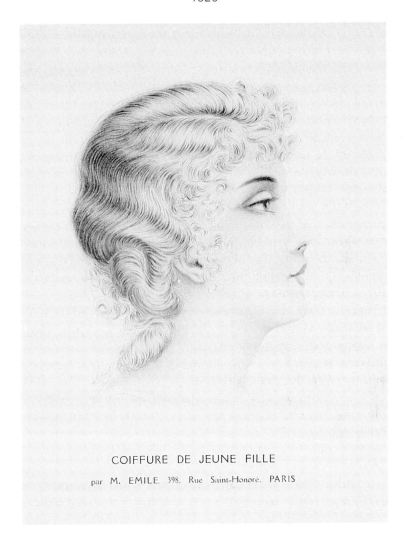

COIFFURE DE JEUNE FILLE

par M. EMILE, 398, Rue Saint-Honoré. PARIS

Figure 37. A fashionable hairstyle for a girl, sketched by M. Emile (Gaston Boudou). From the *Capilartiste*, September 1920.

veil covering them from head to foot and a wreath of white roses on their heads; and the boys in black suits with a wide and deep white brassard on the left arm. Always a great event in family life, people get ready for this religious ceremony a long time beforehand, and so create business generally. The coiffeurs benefit like other traders, curling the hair of both the little ones and their parents, in spite of the objection annually raised to this by the clergy.

Hairdressers, realising the necessity for increasing their incomes, are developing the perfumery sale trade which the big stores took from them. Perceiving that the *clientèle* (principally ladies) did not purchase perfumery when having their hair waved, the coiffeurs became rather concerned, and decided to inform their clients by means of posters – (1) that in order to keep down the prices of saloon work they had added a perfumery department to their business, where all toilet articles could be obtained at the same prices as charged for the same goods at the big stores; (2) that in future they could only give their best attention to those ladies who patronised them for the preparations in question.

The Trade did not have to wait long to reap the results of their offensive. Some clients showed their resentment by taking their custom to other hairdressers, where, however, they were confronted with the same notice. The majority understood that the course outlined was but fair, and they reserved their purchases until visiting their hairdressers, so that they might receive better consideration and service.

It is common knowledge that business affairs have changed since the war. At the wholesale houses, for example, the customer no longer orders his goods with pre-war imperiousness, and nearly everywhere innumerable conditions are imposed upon customers. It is but reasonable, therefore, that the coiffeur, whose trade necessitates much experience and care, should be allowed to impose the solitary condition, so that he may be placed on a level with other workers and business people, and enable him and his family to live with fitting dignity.

July 1920: The Coiffure Seen from Behind

Ladies' hairdressers and master posticheurs are exhibiting numerous wax figures in their windows, which they are frequently turning about in order to show the coiffure in all its aspects. In former times the entrance door was in the middle, and flanked on either side by little show windows; nowadays the shops generally have a door at the side in order to provide for one single but much larger show window, where numerous wax figures and even several pieces of postiche, combs and so forth may be displayed behind the figures.

Not only are wax figures much dearer than they used to be, but the coiffeur can no longer do without having several of them on show; and the more new figures and postiche a shop displays the more business it attracts. This proves that it pays to be progressive, to invest money and reap the many advantages accruing. Those who dissent from this basic principle are wrong, and their competitors benefit by their hesitation and backwardness.

August 1920: The Influence of Hairdressing Exhibitions on the Public

Ladies' hairdressers are so numerous nowadays that they seem to be unable to come to a working arrangement with one another: – (1) The competition involved is of the unhealthy kind, for the simple reason that it is only brought to bear on the question of saloon charges; (2) this state of affairs stands in the way of collective publicity and display, which exert so much influence on the public and in consequence on Fashion.

As regards the first point, I will say but little. Everybody knows that it is a mistaken idea to countenance and foster competition as concerns prices when the question of work is involved. In other business life, it is a different thing entirely; a proprietary article, which may be found everywhere, will certainly be purchased in the cheapest market. But for work done, especially at the ladies' hairdresser's, it is above all individual skill and taste and personal initiative which count in the estimation of the customers. Professional perfection should be the basis of competition amongst coiffeurs, and not saloon charges.

The second point concerns collective publicity display, *i.e.*, exhibitions and demonstrations held for public notice, and which are always of very great importance. If we permit ourselves to glance backwards, we must be astonished at what our predecessors did in order to work up a Fashion to meet their own ends. Two or three decades ago coiffeurs alone possessed wax figures and their displays always caused a furore. It was these attractive exhibitions of hairdressing which gave dressmakers and their prototypes the idea and the desire to follow suit. At the present time the large drapery establishments are in possession of the greatest number of wax figures. Each of these stores possesses about 500, without counting the thousands spread over the establishments of lesser importance and shops of all kinds. All these figures are exhibited in the windows, but their hair is not always dressed by coiffeurs. The best men charge too much, so that the hair is often dressed by improvers, who are not sufficiently experienced, or by people who are not in the Trade, and these do not worry about the superior interests of our profession.

To counterbalance the bad examples shown in the shops of drapers and other traders, the hairdressing fraternity have but a few figures and modest windows in which to show them. If they could afford more outlay for advertising purposes, and, above all, if they understood the urgency of the matter, the coiffeurs might, like their predecessors, organise collective exhibitions, or participate in the great industrial luxury displays, such as that which has scored such a big success in the Jardins des Tuileries. This exhibition lasted for three months and comprised all the luxury trades, except hair-dressing.

There were in this single exhibition over 400 wax figures, each one of which was dressed in a Chinese style so far as the hair was concerned, but superbly robed by the houses which exhibited them. The public were attracted during these three months and, perceiving only Chinese coiffures, many ladies are now persuaded that this fashion is really general. For all these exhibition models are photographed, sketched and described in all the papers.

[Moreover], as a result of the lack of uniformity in the Hairdressing Trade, fashionable ladies are disputing among themselves as regards the *dernière mode*. One lady says to the other, 'I know that the high coiffure is the fashion; if you want to confirm this you will find it on the wax figures of my coiffeur.' The second lady says, 'Not at all. The fashion in hairdressing according to my coiffeur, who knows what he is talking about, is the *coiffure mi-tête*; you can walk round and see his models.' Lastly, the third lady claims that the latest fashion in hairdressing is low, and she likewise gives her reasons. Every fashionable lady has her favourite coiffeur, one in whom she places her confidence, and who to her is always the best coiffeur in the world.

This is all very nice, but it does not solve the problem of a single style which can be set with effective force against the horrible Chinese monstrosities, which will be the ruin of ladies' hairdressers and posticheurs, who are so numerous at the present time.

September 1920: The Slavery of Fashion

I am writing this at a period which it is the custom to call the 'dead' season in Paris and the full season in the watering places. The news which we received from the fashionable sea-side resorts is terrible in regard to the cost of living now ruling in those places and the number of persons who in spite of this are going there.

As for 'restful' holidays, the fashionable ladies live in a state of continual motion – a hundred times more so than even in the Capital. Considering all this at a distance and in quietude one may indulge in a good many pertinent reflections.

For instance, one after another, all trades will soon enjoy the advantages of the short working day (eight hours and perhaps less). Fashionable ladies will alone remain the slaves of their existence, charming though this may be, for fifteen hours per day and perhaps longer still. And this will last eternally, for fashionable ladies will never indulge in a union. From this point of view the coiffeur is in happier circumstances than his aristocratic clients.

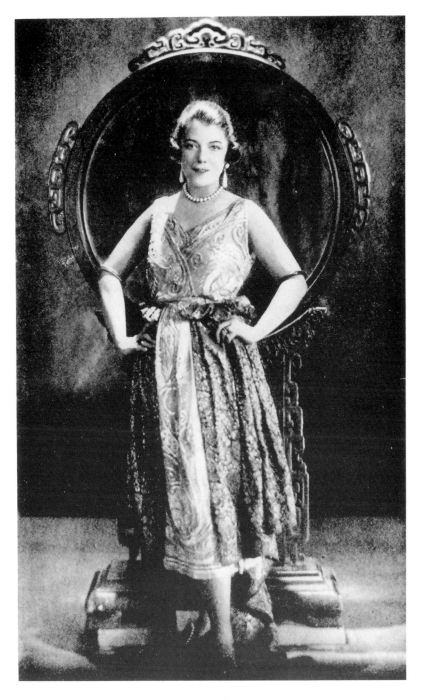

Figure 38. Mlle. Spinelly, one of the era's commanding figures of the stage and high society. From *Vanity Fair*, August 1920.

A ladies' journal published at one of the seaside holiday resorts lays down the dictum that the really fashionable lady must in country life change her dress and coiffure eight times daily: –

(1) The early morning, from nine o'clock: Coiffure with slightly curled fringe in front, softly enveloping the head and with a few curls over the ears. Hair at the nape of the neck fastened by a flat barrette.

(2) At 10 o'clock, ride on horseback: Postiche to imitate cut and waved hair, with parting on the left side. Masculine hat well over the head. Jacket and knickers for riding astride like men.

(3) For dejeuner: Coiffure with the hair taken straight up in front; soft waves on top, finishing at the back of the head in a simple Grecian chignon. The lower part of the coiffure waved and curled.

(4) The hour for bathing: Hair drawn back and hidden under a fancy cap which allows of the use of some small pieces of postiche.

(5) Dinner coiffure: Dressed with a good many fleecy curls around the face; the long hair taken up half high and made into a chignon in the style of a large cravat knot with the ends curled and pendent. Nape of the neck kept free by the use of a large barette.

(6) Ball coiffure: Parting nearly in the middle of the forehead; bandeaux; hair waved in wide undulations; and separated by a band of jewellery. Chignon knotted heavily at the back, rather low, from which protrudes a spray of Paradise plumes.

(7) Lastly the night coiffure, the style of which depends upon the hair, which must be in every case well brushed and carefully combed. Of course a short head of hair can only be left free whilst a medium head of hair is softly raised in a wide roll around a ribbon, which is knotted in fancy style. A long head of hair must be softly plaited to the middle of its length and fastened by a ribbon – no hair pin should remain on the head during the night.

Fashion does not admit of collectivism; on the contrary, it lives and is maintained only by the most independent individualism. It requires, in effect, personal originality, an originality which is ever changing. Certainly there are numerous circles of elegant ladies, but one of these always finishes by emerging from the others. And even in this leading group the ladies of fashion also admit of graduation.

If, therefore, a close investigation were made, it would be possible to discover, by repute, the most fashionable lady of all, in the same manner as it was possible to designate the most beautiful lady in France. But fashion is a sport. And, as in every other sport, fashionable ladies are perpetually competing for the first place. She who attains this glorious goal can only retain it temporarily, and with difficulty, for another aspirant will sooner or later pass her in the race. And so the world rolls on.

The most stupendous efforts are necessary in the world of fashion; the slightest error in taste is in itself sufficient to bring defeat. The price of such a victory is inestimable. The lady who, for the moment, scores a victory is glorified by universal approbation. She is sought after and belauded; her portrait can be seen in the leading journals, together with her biography and the secrets of her success. All of which may be agreeable to the lady herself, but it is done mainly with the object of satisfying the insatiable curiosity of the great public.

People engaged in luxury trades gain their livelihood out of this system of emulation and naturally foster it in every way they can by continually suggesting new ideas and submitting fresh models. Here again, competition is brought into play, and the various tradespeople take part in it with no little zest. A fine advertisement awaits the hairdresser who dresses the hair of the most fashionable queen of the moment. Great efforts are made to this end, and the coiffeur can only hope to attain it by perfecting his professional capabilities and cultivating his judgment and taste.

October 1920: Revival of the Chinese Style of Hairdressing

We have again in our midst an enemy which very soon we shall be no longer able to overcome, so numerous will be its adherents.

Driven from Paris last winter by the energetic counter-attack of the closely allied master hairdressers, the abominable Chinese coiffure has once more made its reappearance this summer at the fashionable French seaside resorts, and threatens seriously to invade the world of fashion.

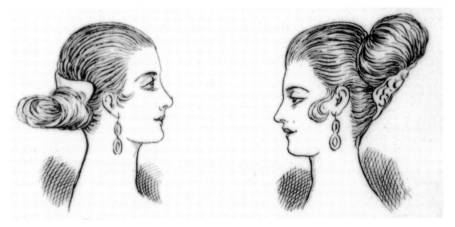

Figure 39. Two versions of the infamous 'Chinese' style. From *HWJS*, October 1920.

A dozen eccentric young ladies caused a sensation at Deauville during the race-meeting week with their hair flattened down and drawn back, and wearing a chignon-coque more or less low and always very conspicuous; their faces made up in 'brunette' style without any *poudre de riz* at all, and consequently high complexioned; with long Oriental pendants from the ears; head and arms bare, and a walking stick in their hands.

In order to exhibit their new coiffure they went about without hats, and attracted considerable notice, if not admiration. Of course, they did not succeed in rallying the majority of their sex to their bad example; but as they are young and pretty, enjoy an aristocratic following, and are in the front rank of society folk – driving superb automobiles during the day and wearing much jewellery in the evening, besides losing fantastic sums at the casino – the crowd follows them and endeavours to copy their example as far as possible.

It is necessary for us to oppose this new style with all our forces, but with discretion, making perhaps here and there a few concessions. Shall we be able once more to emerge triumphant from the struggle, by appealing to the good sense of the public? The Fashion Committee of Paris hopes so, without being able to say definitely. Personally, I estimate that mere persuasion will not be sufficient this time, because the situation is critical. Nobody can tell where this tendency may lead.

Before all else we must learn to know our enemy. What is exactly the most unfavourable form of the new coiffure? It is [that] introduced by Mlle. Diamant, the greatest vedette of the year. Ladies describe it thus: 'The hair entirely brought back and flattened on the head, the hair hanging down behind.' What they call the 'piece of hair hanging down the back' is the long chignon which is held by a single comb without any hair pins. Evidently this long chignon and the bringing of the hair over the forehead give to the feminine head an appearance to which we are not accustomed.

Noticing with misgiving that his clients are one after the other abandoning waving and fluffy coiffures, a ladies' hairdresser at Deauville, M. Caloun, who employs twenty-seven assistants during the season, made a proposal to all those ladies who wished him to dress their hair in the 'fashionable Chinese style.' His idea was entertained by quite a number who decided to try it. It is rather less straight than [Mlle. Diamant's], and comprises, beyond the hair in front of the ears, a large coque chignon and a nice comb. The large coque chignon is very easy to obtain with a small piece of false hair, and by its use the coiffeur made a good thing out of the chinese coiffures. He sold more than two hundred pieces of hair and as many large carved combs in two weeks at an average price of 150 francs. That was clearly a more intelligent attitude to adopt than simply but persistently to grumble about the fashion.

November 1920: Paris Hairdressing Style

The same evening as the great historical hairdressing competition took place in Brussels, a similar event was being held in Paris with the double object of celebrating the 100th anniversary of our Mutual Aid Society, St. Louis et Union, and the reopening of its school classes.

It was in every respect a very fine event, but I shall only refer to it here from the hairdressing point of view.

Thirty professors executed about sixty head-dresses, half of which were historical or allegorical coiffures, and the rest evening coiffures. There were seven historical or allegorical coiffures which received money prizes: – (1) Transformation in grey hair by M. Lazartigues (150 francs); (2) 'Déjeuner d'oiseaux,' a white coiffure ornamented with cherries, by M. Dutrait (100 francs); (3) 'Bergère Watteau,' by M. Lechapt (100 francs); (4) 'Merveilleuse Consulat,' by M. Manson (50 francs); (5) 'Coiffure 1830,' by M. Manson (50 francs); (6) 'Marquise Louis XV,' by M. Conet (25 francs); (7) 'Marie Antoinette,' by M. Barraud (25 francs).

Amongst the travesty [i.e., fantasy] coiffures, which were not awarded prizes, there were also some fine examples of expert execution and even a few original ideas. I will mention only the coiffures by M. Antoine, the young leader of our Parisian modernists, which were executed in the ancient Egyptian style and ornamented with a multitude of small plaits of red, blue and green and other coloured hair. These ornaments of hair in unusual colours seem as if they are becoming the fashion, in very many varieties of head ornaments, imitating ropes, ribbons, stuffs, fringes, flowers, etc. The originality and success depend on the imagination and skill of the coiffeur in handling them.

December 1920: A Variety of Evening Coiffures to Counteract the Chinese Styles

As the present rate of exchange is for the time being favourable to the majority of France's neighbours, Paris has recently been visited by a large number of foreign hairdressers. During the day these confrères from other countries have visited our capital, and made their purchases; in the evening we took them to our soirées or they entertained us at the theatre.

At our Trade soirées old friends are to be met, with whom one is always happy to talk 'shop,' and witness the efforts of the younger members of the Trade to improve in waving and dressing in order to construct academic coiffures which are often very complicated, and generally rather stiff and rigid in appearance.

The theatre is much more entertaining: there are always plenty of people present, and one has time to look round and observe, the auditorium and the stage being both available for this purpose. The first statement which may be made is this: Whilst individually everybody is complaining of the hard times, and the difficulties of business, the theatres are full in spite of the exorbitant prices charged for seats. Taken as a whole, an enormous amount of luxury is always in evidence. Extravagant expenditure is continuous; if it is not one set of people, it is the other, whilst fashions become more and more gorgeous. People really seem not to know what to devise in order to incur useless expenditure, but all they undertake with this idea in view is sure to be effective.

The libertine pieces which are played on the Parisian stage are always fairly numerous, and no expense is spared in the luxurious nature of the decorations and toilettes. There may be seen handsome women, gorgeous costumes, and a few original and audacious coiffures, [reflecting] the eclecticism which is predominant at the present time amongst fashionable ladies in Paris.

Besides the coiffures dressed low, flat or half-high, we have also notices several raised coiffures, which were worn especially by short ladies. These high coiffures when properly executed are not yet out of fashion for evening wear, and for all ordinary occasions. Nevertheless, it is so difficult to execute the fashionable high coiffures properly, and especially to make them last a certain time in good condition, that postiche is often resorted to.

In short, if the variety of the coiffures has an attraction for spectators, it is also necessary that the hair should be clean, brilliant and nicely arranged, without too many complications.

Index